Clinical Guide to
DEPRESSION and
BIPOLAR DISORDER

Findings From the
COLLABORATIVE DEPRESSION
STUDY

Clinical Guide to
DEPRESSION and
BIPOLAR DISORDER
Findings From the
COLLABORATIVE DEPRESSION
STUDY

Editor-in-Chief

Martin B. Keller, M.D.

Co-editors

William H. Coryell, M.D.
Jean Endicott, Ph.D.
Jack D. Maser, Ph.D.
Pamela J. Schettler, Ph.D.

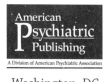

American Psychiatric Publishing
A Division of American Psychiatric Association

Washington, DC
London, England

Note: The authors have worked to ensure that all information in this book is accurate at the time of publication and consistent with general psychiatric and medical standards, and that information concerning drug dosages, schedules, and routes of administration is accurate at the time of publication and consistent with standards set by the U.S. Food and Drug Administration and the general medical community. As medical research and practice continue to advance, however, therapeutic standards may change. Moreover, specific situations may require a specific therapeutic response not included in this book. For these reasons and because human and mechanical errors sometimes occur, we recommend that readers follow the advice of physicians directly involved in their care or the care of a member of their family.

Books published by American Psychiatric Publishing (APP) represent the findings, conclusions, and views of the individual authors and do not necessarily represent the policies and opinions of APP or the American Psychiatric Association.

If you would like to buy between 25 and 99 copies of this or any other American Psychiatric Publishing title, you are eligible for a 20% discount; please contact Customer Service at appi@psych.org or 800-368-5777. If you wish to buy 100 or more copies of the same title, please e-mail us at bulksales@psych.org for a price quote.

Copyright © 2013 American Psychiatric Association
ALL RIGHTS RESERVED

Manufactured in the United States of America on acid-free paper
17   16   15   14   13   5   4   3   2   1
First Edition

Typeset in Adobe's Chaparral Pro and Frutiger LT Std.

American Psychiatric Publishing,
a Division of American Psychiatric Association
1000 Wilson Boulevard
Arlington, VA 22209-3901
www.appi.org

Library of Congress Cataloging-in-Publication Data
Clinical guide to depression and bipolar disorder : findings from the Collaborative Depression Study / editor-in-chief, Martin B. Keller ; co-editors, William H. Coryell ... [et al.]. — 1st ed.
      p. ; cm.
   Includes bibliographical references and index.
   ISBN 978-1-58562-433-1 (pbk. : alk. paper)
   I. Keller, Martin B. II. American Psychiatric Association.
   [DNLM: 1. Collaborative Depression Study. 2. Depressive Disorder—United States. 3. Bipolar Disorder—United States. 4. Clinical Trials as Topic—United States. WM 171.5]
   RC537
   616.85′27—dc23

                                                             2013005966

British Library Cataloguing in Publication Data
A CIP record is available from the British Library.

Contents

Contributors

Hagop S. Akiskal, M.D.
Distinguished Professor of Psychiatry, Department of Psychiatry, University of California, San Diego

Robert Boland, M.D.
Professor, Department of Psychiatry and Human Behavior, Alpert Medical School, Brown University, Providence, Rhode Island

Paula Clayton, M.D.
Medical Director, American Foundation for Suicide Prevention, New York, New York

William H. Coryell, M.D.
Professor, Department of Psychiatry, University of Iowa, Carver College of Medicine, Iowa City, Iowa

Jean Endicott, Ph.D.
Professor of Clinical Psychology, Department of Psychiatry, College of Physicians and Surgeons, Columbia University, New York, New York; Director, Division of Clinical Phenomenology, New York State Psychiatric Institute, New York, New York

Jan A. Fawcett, M.D.
Professor, Department of Psychiatry, University of New Mexico, Albuquerque, New Mexico

Jess G. Fiedorowicz, M.D., Ph.D.
Assistant Professor, Department of Psychiatry, Department of Internal Medicine, Carver College of Medicine; Department of Epidemiology, College of Public Health, The University of Iowa, Iowa City

Deborah Hasin, Ph.D.
Professor of Clinical Epidemiology (in Psychiatry), Departments of Epidemiology and Psychiatry, Columbia University, New York, New York; New York State Psychiatric Institute, New York, New York

Robert M.A. Hirschfeld, M.D.
Titus H. Harris Chair and Harry K. Davis Professor, Professor and Chair, Department of Psychiatry, The University of Texas Medical Branch, Galveston, Texas

Lewis L. Judd, M.D.
Mary Gilman Marston Professor, Distinguished Professor and Chair, Department of Psychiatry, University of California, San Diego

Martin B. Keller, M.D.
Professor, Department of Psychiatry and Human Behavior, Alpert Medical School, Brown University; Chief Academic Strategic Planning and Director, Mood and Anxiety Disorders Research Program, Butler Hospital, Providence, Rhode Island

Bari Kilcoyne, B.S.
Graduate Student, Department of Epidemiology, Columbia University, New York, New York

Andrew Leon, Ph.D.
Professor of Public Health and of Biostatistics in Psychiatry, Weill Cornell Medical College, New York, New York (deceased)

Chunshan Li, M.A.
Research Biostatistician, Weill Medical College of Cornell University, New York, N.Y.

Jack D. Maser, Ph.D.
Formerly at the National Institute of Mental Health and Adjunct Professor, Department of Psychiatry, University of California, San Diego (retired)

John P. Rice, Ph.D.
Professor of Mathematics in Psychiatry, Department of Psychiatry, Washington University School of Medicine, St. Louis, Missouri

Pamela J. Schettler, Ph.D.
Senior Statistician, Department of Psychiatry, University of California, San Diego; Senior Research Associate, Department of Psychiatry and Behavioral Sciences, Emory University, Atlanta, Georgia

David Solomon, M.D.
Clinical Associate Professor, Department of Psychiatry and Human Behavior, Alpert Medical School, Brown University; Deputy Editor of Psychiatry, UpToDate

Disclosure of Interests

The following contributors to this book have indicated a financial interest in or other affiliation with a commercial supporter, a manufacturer of a commercial product, a provider of a commercial service, a nongovernmental organization, and/ or a government agency, as listed below:

Robert M. A. Hirschfeld, M.D.—*Continuing medical education:* CME Outfitters, Letters & Sciences, Nevada Psychiatric Association. *Honorarium:* Service on *Merck Manual* editorial board. *Royalties:* Jones and Bartlett.
Martin B. Keller, M.D.—*Advisory board:* CeNeRx BioPharma. *Consulting/ Honoraria:* CeNeRx BioPharma, Medtronic, Sierra Neuropharmaceuticals. *Grants/research:* Pfizer.
Andrew Leon, Ph.D.— *Consulting/Advising:* MedAvante, Roche, National Institute of Mental Health, U.S. Food and Drug Administration. *Membership on independent boards monitoring data and safety:* AstraZeneca, Pfizer, Sunovion. *Equity:* MedAvante.
Pamela J. Schettler, Ph.D.—*Statistical consulting:* BrainCells Inc., Cedars-Sinai Medical Center, MSI Methylation Sciences, Inc., Partners HealthCare (Massachusetts General Hospital).
David Solomon, M.D.—*Editorship:* Deputy Editor for Psychiatry, UpToDate, Wolters Kluwer Health.

The following contributors have indicated that they have no financial interests or other affiliations that represent or could appear to represent a competing interest with their contributions to this book:

Hagop S. Akiskal, M.D.; Robert J. Boland, M.D.; William H. Coryell, M.D.; Jean Endicott, Ph.D.; Jan A. Fawcett, M.D.; Jess G. Fiedorowicz, M.D., Ph.D.; Deborah Hasin, Ph.D.; Lewis L. Judd, M.D.; Bari Kilcoyne, B.S.; Chunsan Li, M.A.; Jack D. Maser, Ph.D.; John P. Rice, Ph.D.

Dedication

THE COLLABORATIVE Depression Study (CDS) was conceptualized by several individuals in the early 1970s. Their vision of a study on the phenomenology, diagnosis, genetics, and longitudinal clinical course of depression influenced research and practice for decades. Originators of the CDS included Martin M. Katz, Ph.D., Gerald Klerman, M.D., Eli Robins, M.D., Robert L. Spitzer, M.D., and George Winokur, M.D. We dedicate this volume to these men, three of whom are deceased. Highlights of their extraordinary careers are summarized later in this dedication.

In addition to the originators listed in the previous paragraph and the authors of the chapters included in this book, many investigators have been involved in the CDS, including Nancy Andreasen, M.D., David Clarke, Ph.D., Jack Croughan, M.D., Robert Gibbons, Ph.D., Philip Lavori, Ph.D., Andrew Leon, Ph.D. (deceased), Patricia McDonald-Scott, M.A., Timothy Muller, M.D., Theodore Reich, M.D. (deceased), M. Tracie Shea, Ph.D., William Scheftner, M.D., Robert Shapiro, M.D. (deceased), Amos Wellner, M.D., and Michael Young, Ph.D. We are extremely grateful for their contributions to the CDS.

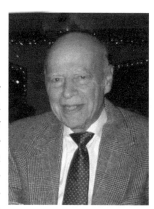

Martin M. Katz, Ph.D.

Martin M. Katz received his Ph.D. in Psychology and Physiology from the University of Texas in 1955 and subsequently served as a staff member in the Psychopharmacology Branch at the National Institute of Mental Health (NIMH). In 1968, he was appointed Chief of the Clinical Research Branch at the NIMH. In that role, he organized and supported the national conferences on research that resulted in the development of the CDS.

After retiring from the NIMH, Dr. Katz served as a faculty member at the Albert Einstein College of Medicine in New York City and the Department of Psychiatry at the University of Texas Health Science Center in San Antonio. In addition, Dr. Katz has been an active consultant to the Mental Health Division at the World Health Organization for many years. He is the author of more than 100 scientific publications on the phenomenology of depression and on the relation of antidepressants to specific behaviors. He developed several clinical instruments—most notably, the Katz Adjustment Scales.

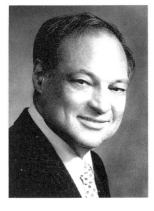

Gerald Klerman, M.D.

Gerald Klerman, M.D., a native of New York, received his medical degree from New York University School of Medicine and trained in psychiatry at Bellevue Hospital and at Massachusetts Mental Health Center at Harvard Medical School. Dr. Klerman served on the faculties of Harvard Medical School and Yale University. In 1970, he became the superintendent of the Erich Lindemann Mental Health Center and professor of psychiatry at Harvard Medical School.

He was appointed to the position of administrator of the Alcohol, Drug Abuse, and Mental Health Administration of the Public Health Service and U.S. Department of Health and Human Services in 1977, where he served until 1980. He subsequently returned to Harvard until he was recruited to become professor and associate chair for research in the Department of Psychiatry at Cornell University Medical College in 1985, where he served until his death in 1992.

Dr. Klerman was one of the most well known and influential psychiatrists of the twentieth century. His work related to nearly every aspect of psychiatry, particularly diagnosis and classification, epidemiology, pharmacotherapy, and psychotherapy (with his wife, Myrna Weissman, Ph.D., who served as a co-developer of interpersonal therapy, a brief psychotherapy for ambulatory depressed patients).

Eli Robins, M.D.

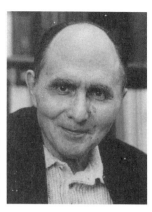

Eli Robins, M.D., a native of Texas, received his medical degree from Harvard Medical School and subsequently trained in psychiatry and neurology at the Massachusetts General Hospital, at McLean Hospital, and at Pratt Diagnostic Hospital. He then joined the faculty at Washington University in St. Louis, Missouri, where he was appointed to chair in 1963. He died in 1994.

Dr. Robins was a "pivotal player in establishing American psychiatry as a scientific discipline" (R. E. Hudgens and G. E. Murphy, *Archives of General Psychiatry,* 52:1080–1081, 1995). In the mid-twentieth century, American psychiatric thinking was dominated by psychodynamic and psychoanalytic theory. With his colleagues, Lee Robins, Ph.D. (his wife), Samuel Guze, M.D., and George Winokur, M.D., he challenged this theory and promoted an empirical approach to psychiatric illness, emphasizing objective observations, follow-up, and family studies. With his collaborators at Washington University, he developed the Feighner criteria that formed the basis for DSM-III and transformed the approach to diagnosis in the United States and the world.

Robert L. Spitzer, M.D.

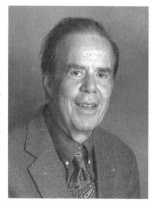

Robert L. Spitzer, M.D., a native of New York, received his medical degree from New York University School of Medicine and trained in psychiatry at Columbia University. He then joined the faculty at Columbia and remained there until his retirement.

Dr. Spitzer made seminal contributions to clinical instrumentation and approach to diagnosis. Along with his colleague Jean Endicott, Ph.D., as well as with Janet Williams, D.S.W., Miriam Gibbon, M.S.W., and Michael B. First, M.D., he developed clinical interviews, the Schedule for Affective Disorders and Schizophrenia (SADS), and the Structured Clinical Interview for DSM Disorders (SCID). Dr. Spitzer chaired the DSM-III and DSM-III-R work groups for the American Psychiatric Association, which represented a major shift in the approach to diagnosis in psychiatry in the United States.

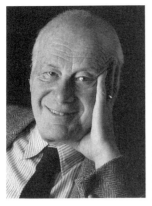

George Winokur, M.D.

George Winokur, M.D., a native of Philadelphia, Pennsylvania, received his medical degree from the University of Maryland. He subsequently served on the faculty at Washington University School of Medicine before becoming the head of the Department of Psychiatry at the University of Iowa in 1971, a position that he held until 1990. He continued his work until his death in 1996.

His collaborations with Eli Robins, M.D., and Samuel Guze, M.D., involved the first diagnostic criteria based on operationally defined variables to come into wide use. As previously noted, this system became the basis for DSM-III. Dr. Winokur made seminal contributions to family studies in mood disorders. He also made contributions to our understanding of the long-term course of depression and schizophrenia through his work on the Iowa 500 Study and the CDS.

CHAPTER 1

Introduction

Robert M. A. Hirschfeld, M.D.
Jack D. Maser, Ph.D.
Martin B. Keller, M.D.

THE NATIONAL INSTITUTE of Mental Health (NIMH) Collaborative Program on the Psychobiology of Depression (now referred to as the *Collaborative Depression Study,* or CDS) has its roots in the 1950s and 1960s. During this period, descriptive psychiatry and biological psychiatry were emerging and becoming influential in the United States, challenging psychodynamic psychiatry, which represented the prevailing approach in psychiatry. The challenge and controversy revolved around the nature and treatment of depression. Many experts believed that there was a pathophysiological basis for depression and that the mechanism of action of the recently introduced antidepressant drugs could be explained in ways consistent with the current theory in this area. The pathophysiological basis for depression was explained primarily by the catecholamine hypothesis, which had been proffered by Schildkraut (1965), Bunney and Davis (1965), and Goodwin et al. (1970) (Hirschfeld 2000). In essence, some depressions were thought to be caused by a deficiency of brain catecholamines, particularly norepinephrine. Elation, a prime diagnostic indicator of mania, was thought to be caused by an excess of such amines (Schildkraut 1965).

The putative mechanism of action of antidepressants supported the catecholamine hypothesis in the following manner. Some patients with tuberculosis being treated by iproniazid, a monoamine oxidase inhibitor, showed

1

improved mood. Studies with reserpine in the 1950s also supported the hypothesis (Carlsson et al. 1957; Muller et al. 1955; Shore et al. 1955). Reserpine interferes with vesicular storage of both serotonin and norepinephrine, thereby depleting presynaptic levels of monoamines available for synaptic release. Clinically, these studies found that reserpine, which causes a reduction in catecholamines, produced severe depressions in some patients (Achor et al. 1955; Harris 1957; Muller et al. 1955). At about the same time, Herting et al. (1961) reported that imipramine, an antidepressant that does not inhibit monoamine oxidase, interfered with the reuptake of norepinephrine into afferent neurons. In addition, Strom-Olsen and Weil-Malherbe (1958) reported that metabolites of norepinephrine were decreased in the urine of patients with depression and increased during mania, suggesting a link between norepinephrine levels and mood.

The role of serotonin in the pathophysiology of mood disorders was based on several observations made during the 1950s. At that time, it was reported that the hallucinogen LSD (lysergic acid diethylamide) blocked serotonin receptors in the brain (Woolley and Shaw 1954), and Gaddum (1963) suggested that serotonin might have a role in the etiology of mood disorders. Shore and others (1955) noted that reserpine depleted brain serotonin stores (in addition to norepinephrine stores) and increased concentrations of the serotonin metabolite 5-hydroxyindoleacetic acid (5-HIAA) in urine. On the basis of a series of empirical findings, Aghajanian and co-workers (1968, 1970; Haigler and Aghajanian 1973) suggested the operation of a negative feedback regulatory mechanism such that raphe electrical activity decreases (presumably with a corresponding depression of serotonin synthesis) when the postsynaptic neuron signals the presence of excess serotonin. Maser et al. (1975) then examined a behavior in the whole animal and essentially replicated the neuronal findings by observing increases or decreases in tonic immobility, depending on the nature of a compound's action on serotonin.

Confirmation of the role of monoamines in the pathophysiology of depression and the mechanism of antidepressants was thwarted by several factors. First, great controversy existed about how to classify depressions, limiting the ability of biological researchers to identify those depressions that likely had a pathophysiological basis. Among the approaches to the diagnosis of depression at that time were the endogenous/reactive distinction, the primary/secondary distinction, the bipolar/unipolar distinction, and the psychotic/neurotic distinction. Furthermore, even if the researchers knew which distinction to use, no good clinical assessment techniques were available to gather clinical information; reliable and valid diagnostic criteria sets for the different subcategories of mood disorders also were not available.

Another limitation faced by biological researchers was that the biological findings resulted from small studies, limiting generalizability and replicability. In addition, no standardized methods for conducting bioassays were accepted and used by the field.

Epidemiological Findings Underscoring the Importance of the Collaborative Depression Study

Another major collaborative research study was initiated by the NIMH shortly after the inception of the CDS: the Epidemiologic Catchment Area (ECA) Study (Eaton et al. 1981). The ECA Study found that depression was much more prevalent than had been thought (Blazer et al. 1988). Prior to the ECA Study, psychiatric epidemiology was very limited and beset by problems similar to those of the early biological studies: earlier DSM editions were neither criterion based nor descriptive, and no standardized, structured interviews were available to elicit the data. As a result, diagnosticians had poor interrater reliability.

The ECA Study was planned to include well-trained interviewers; standardized assessments geared to DSM-III (American Psychiatric Association 1980) criteria; and a stratified, national, randomized sample. The data indicated a lifetime prevalence for any affective disorder of 8.3% of the population and a 1-month (or point) prevalence of 5.2. The subsequent National Comorbidity Survey adjusted that number upward by reporting that 17.1% of adults had a lifetime form of depression (Blazer et al. 1994). Reanalysis of ECA bipolar symptoms from a spectrum perspective yielded a 6.4% lifetime prevalence for the bipolar spectrum, consisting of manic, hypomanic, and subsyndromal manic symptoms (Judd and Akiskal 2003).

A major problem, however, was that DSM-III had rather rigid boundaries around its disorders such that when comorbidity was present—and it almost always was—depression was counted when criteria were met for depression and other disorders, such as anxiety. When criteria for an anxiety disorder were met and depression was present, each disorder was diagnosed as a separate category when, in fact, they were mixed. Mixed depression and anxiety and mixed depression and bipolarity yielded increased prevalence numbers (Clayton 1990; Zinbarg et al. 1994). Moreover, the spectrum concept had been growing and slowly undercutting the categorical format traditionally used in DSM (for reviews, see Maser and Akiskal 2002; Cassano et al. 1997). In Chapter 15, "Impact of Anxiety Severity on Mood Disorders," Fawcett et al. provide an up-to-date review of how the spectrum concept is currently influencing DSM-5.

In terms of functional impairment, based on a U.S. population of 300,000,000, ECA data suggest that almost 25 million U.S. citizens are depressed sometime over their lifetime, and the National Comorbidity Survey data raise that number dramatically to 51.3 million (Kessler et al. 1996; Regier et al. 1978), or slightly more than 16% of the U.S. population. Recently, depression was documented as the third leading cause of disability-adjusted life-years among all ages worldwide (World Health Organization 2004). These are highly significant and disturbing numbers given that treatment possibilities are plentiful and varied, though often inaccessible.

It is important not to overgeneralize the epidemiological findings and acknowledge that a meaningful proportion of patients with major depressive disorder (MDD) or bipolar disorder experience only a single lifetime episode. For many, however, chronicity, frequent recurrence, and the pervasiveness of the resulting disability make mood disorders an enormous public health problem.

Inception of the Collaborative Program on the Psychobiology of Depression

The excitement about the theories of the pathophysiology of depression and the mechanism of action of antidepressant medications led the NIMH to organize a major conference on the psychobiology of depression in 1969. The aims of that conference were to seek an up-to-date analysis of current research, identify obstacles to progress, and consider potential solutions that might accelerate the pace of research in the field (Katz et al. 1979). Following the conference, the participants recommended that an intensive research effort be undertaken to focus on three main areas:

1. *Nosology*—the development of a sound, reliable system of classification of the depressive disorders.
2. *Genetics*—the design of studies to permit the definitive test of hypotheses concerning the role of genetics.
3. *Pathophysiology*—the investigation of the role of specific biochemical, neurophysiological, and endocrine mechanisms implicated in the etiology of depression.

Biological Studies

An advisory committee on the psychobiology of depression under the leadership of Martin Katz, Ph.D., was established in 1971 to help implement these recommendations. Out of this work came the first component of the NIMH CDS—namely, the *biological studies* component (Katz et al. 1979). The biological studies component had two important features that would make it unique

TABLE 1–1. Initiating investigators and participating centers of the National Institute of Mental Health (NIMH) Clinical Research Branch Collaborative Program on the Psychobiology of Depression: biological studies component

James Maas, M.D., Chair

Investigators	Institution
John Davis, M.D.; David Garver, M.D.	Illinois State Psychiatric Institute
James Maas, M.D.; Eugene Redmond, M.D.	Yale University
Joe Mendels, M.D.; Allan Ramsey, M.D.	Philadelphia VA Hospital, University of Pennsylvania
Eli Robins, M.D.; Amos Weiner, M.D.	Washington University
Peter Stokes, M.D.; James Kocsis, M.D.	Cornell University
Martin Katz, Ph.D.; Steven Secunda, M.D.; Stephen Koslow, Ph.D.[a]	NIMH

[a]Coordinator.

and hopefully definitive in terms of testing the catecholamine hypothesis. First, it included a large sample of carefully characterized patients. Second, the study allowed simultaneous assessment of neurotransmitter, neuroendocrine, and electrolyte systems, permitting examination of correlations among these systems and their relations with behavioral and clinical factors. Simultaneous assessment of these relations had never been done. All patients would be interviewed with standardized assessment techniques and given diagnoses based on operationalized criteria.

The study was led by scientists from five major university hospitals (Katz et al. 1979; Maas et al. 1980), and the NIMH staff coordinator was Stephen Koslow, Ph.D. (Table 1–1). Nearly 350 psychiatric inpatients with unipolar depression, bipolar depression, mania, or several control conditions received careful diagnostic assessment and measurement of electrolyte metabolism, biogenic amine disposition, and neuroendocrine function. Cerebrospinal fluid, blood, and urine samples were taken, and some of these measures were repeated weekly.

Clinical Studies

The *clinical studies* component of the CDS was developed to complement the biological studies component. New diagnostic and assessment instruments were used to describe subjects' history, intake characteristics, and follow-up course (Katz et al. 1979). The aims of the clinical studies component were to address nosological, genetic, and psychosocial issues with regard to affective disorders:

- To resolve certain current issues of nosology through a comparative analysis of the major extant classification systems for affective disorders.
- To test current prominent and novel genetic hypotheses.
- To investigate the role of psychosocial factors such as personality and environment in the nature and maintenance of depressive states.

Gerald Klerman, M.D., and Martin Katz, Ph.D., served as chairs, and Robert M.A. Hirschfeld, M.D., was the original NIMH coordinator. Hirschfeld subsequently became the project director and co-chairman of the study. When Gerald Klerman left Harvard University in early 1977 to become the administrator of the Alcohol, Drug Abuse, and Mental Health Administration, Martin B. Keller, M.D., took over as principal investigator at the Massachusetts General Hospital site. When Klerman returned to Harvard in 1980, his involvement in the study was substantially diminished. This and Hirschfeld's departure from the NIMH in 1990 to the University of Texas Medical Branch left a dearth in leadership in the CDS. In response, Keller stepped forward and assumed leadership of the group as chair of the steering committee, with William H. Coryell, M,D., as co-chair and Jack D. Maser, Ph.D., as NIMH staff coordinator. Under Keller's tutelage, the study evolved from one of primarily studying nosology to a comprehensive short interview interval, prospective, observational follow-up extended to more than 30 years that provided invaluable data on the effect of mood disorders on people's lives.

The development of a standardized clinical interview and set of clear and reproducible diagnostic criteria were needed to address the major aims of the CDS. The results were the Schedule for Affective Disorders and Schizophrenia (SADS; Endicott and Spitzer 1978) and the Research Diagnostic Criteria (RDC; Spitzer et al. 1978). The SADS is an interview guide and recording document for information about a subject's functioning and manifest symptomatology. Different versions of the SADS were developed for use with relatives, control subjects, and specialized evaluations, as described in the Chapter 2, "Collaborative Depression Study Procedures and Study Design," in this volume. The RDC—a modification and elaboration of some of the diagnostic criteria referred to as the Feighner criteria (Feighner et al. 1972), which had been developed at Washington University Department of Psychiatry—comprises a set of operational, precisely defined criteria for functional psychiatric disorders with a focus primarily on affective disorders (Spitzer et al. 1978). An indication of the early effect of the CDS and its investigators is DSM-III. DSM-

III was based on the RDC and was a major departure from prior official nomenclatures in that it focused on observable clinical characteristics and history, not on inferred etiological beliefs.

In addition, a set of measures to assess life events, the Psychiatric Epidemiology Research Interview–Modified (Hirschfeld et al. 1977b) and a measure of interpersonal dependency, were developed (Hirschfeld et al. 1977a). Undue interpersonal dependency was believed to be the personality precursor to depression in the psychodynamic and psychoanalytic literature (Chodoff 1973).

In 1974, a pilot program involving 150 moderately to severely depressed patients was undertaken at four major university centers to perform a field trial for the SADS and the RDC, as well as a feasibility study for other measures (Endicott and Spitzer 1979). The pilot study went very well, with reliabilities of symptoms on the SADS between 0.82 and 0.99 (Endicott and Spitzer 1978) and diagnostic test-retest reliabilities ranging from 0.49 to 0.93 (Spitzer et al. 1978).

In 1977, the actual clinical studies component was initiated (Katz et al. 1979) involving five teaching hospitals, four of which had conducted the pilot study: Massachusetts General Hospital, Harvard Medical School, Boston; Rush-Presbyterian-St. Luke's Hospital, Rush College of Medicine, Chicago, Illinois; University of Iowa College of Medicine, Iowa City; New York State Psychiatric Institute, Columbia University College of Physicians and Surgeons, New York; and Washington University School of Medicine, St. Louis, Missouri (Table 1–2). The protocol included 955 probands and 2,225 relatives.

Of the 955 probands, 616 were expected to participate in a family study. Although the mood disorders, including depression and bipolar disorder, were the major inclusion criteria, probands entered the study with a host of coexisting disorders (see Chapter 2). Spouses and first-degree relatives were assessed for psychopathology with the Lifetime version of the SADS (SADS-L). No attempt was made to control or prescribe treatment, and outside of the research assessments, subjects proceeded through the clinical workup, treatment, and follow-up with their clinicians in the usual way. Thus, the study design was prospective, longitudinal, and naturalistic.

Transformation of the Collaborative Depression Study Into an Extended Longitudinal Study

In the original protocol, patients were to be followed up for 2 years. However, the pilot data were sufficiently exciting that the investigators, the peer review panel, and the NIMH realized that an extended study of the diverse aspects of depres-

TABLE 1–2. Initiating investigators and participating centers of the National Institute of Mental Health (NIMH) Clinical Research Branch Collaborative Program on the Psychobiology of Depression: clinical studies component

Gerald Klerman, M.D., and Martin Katz, Ph.D., Chairmen

Investigators	Institution
Gerald Klerman, M.D.; Robert Shapiro, M.D.; Martin Keller, M.D.	Massachusetts General Hospital, Harvard Medical School
Jan Fawcett, M.D.; William Scheftner, M.D.	Rush-Presbyterian-St Luke's Hospital
George Winokur, M.D.; Nancy Andreasen, M.D.	University of Iowa
Robert L. Spitzer, M.D.; Jean Endicott, M.D.	New York State Psychiatric Institute
Eli Robins, M.D.; Paula Clayton, M.D.; Theodore Reich, M.D.; Amos Weiner, M.D.	Washington University School of Medicine
Martin Katz, Ph.D.; Robert Hirschfeld, M.D.[a]	NIMH

[a]Coordinator.

sion should be planned. Early results of the CDS documented a clinical course of depression much worse than had been described previously: episode durations were longer, and relapse and recurrence rates were higher, as were rates of chronicity. These stunning findings spurred the investigators to change the aims of the CDS to investigate the long-term course of affective disorders. Through various funding increments, the CDS eventually went on to interview participants at 6-month intervals for the first 5 years of follow-up and yearly thereafter for up to 31 years. The development of the aims, hypotheses, and assessments for the new comprehensive prospective, observational, long-term follow-up of the course of the probands in the CDS was conceptualized by Keller and Robert Shapiro, M.D., in collaboration with Jean Endicott, Ph.D., and Robert Spitzer, M.D., aided by many other CDS investigators and directed by Keller after Shapiro's death in 1980. The follow-up assessments were conducted with the Longitudinal Interval Follow-up Evaluation (LIFE), as developed by Keller et al. (1987), and other follow-up instruments, which are described in detail in Chapter 2.

    Thus, the scope of the CDS developed into a unique longitudinal study as the basis for a more comprehensive description of the multiple aspects of the

affective disorders, validation of alternative classification systems and nosological classes, study of family and genetic factors, and exploration of the role
of psychosocial stressors and personality in the symptom manifestations and
clinical course of affective disorders.

Topics Covered in This Book

In choosing the chapters for this book, we had to be selective, given the enormous number of peer-reviewed publications from the CDS. We begin with a
detailed review of the assessments, procedures, and study design in Chapter 2,
almost all of which were designed for the CDS by its collaborators and, in and
of themselves, represented major advances in the field's ability to assess multiple domains of psychopathology, functioning, and treatment. Most of these
measures and methods are still in use today, and the unique design of the follow-up methods has been used in more than 1,000 research studies worldwide. For example, the National Institute of Neurological Disorders and
Stroke (NINDS) included the CDS follow-up instrument (LIFE; Keller et al.
1987) in the Common Data Element Project, a repository of tools for investigators to use when conducting clinical research. This repository will be acces-
sible to the working groups of the NINDS and for public use.

The next two chapters present a dimensional approach to the study of
symptom severity in unipolar MDD (Chapter 3, "Dimensional Symptomatic
Structure of the Long-Term Course of Unipolar Major Depressive Disorder")
and bipolar disorders (Chapter 4, "Dimensional Symptomatic Structure of the
Long-Term Course of Bipolar I and Bipolar II Disorders"). Four affective symptom severity levels are defined according to weekly psychiatric status on all affective conditions: symptoms meeting the diagnostic threshold for major
affective episodes (major depressive episode and mania), symptoms meeting
the diagnostic threshold for lesser affective episodes (minor or intermittent
depression, dysthymia, or hypomania), subsyndromal symptoms below the
threshold for major or minor affective syndromes, and the asymptomatic status (absence of all affective symptoms). Patients experience these affective
symptom severity levels in a dynamic and fluctuating manner during their
long-term course of illness, even within affective episodes. CDS findings based
on the dimensional analysis of symptom severity are presented on the topics of
chronicity, predominance of symptoms below the threshold for MDD and mania, predominance of depressive over manic or hypomanic symptoms in bipolar I and bipolar II disorders, changes in psychosocial impairment associated
with stepwise changes in symptom severity level within subjects, and the importance of resolution of residual symptoms for achieving true episode recovery. Analyses based on the dimensional approach show the true longitudinal

symptomatic nature of major affective disorders. Implications for the clinical management of these disorders are presented based on the findings.

The CDS prospectively observed 39 suicides and many more suicide attempts covering a spectrum of seriousness. In Chapter 5, "Risk Factors for Suicide Attempts and Completions," Coryell describes the risk factors, including the symptoms and temperament measures that proved the most consistent for attempts and completions, in both the short and the long term. The review also covers the ongoing relations between antidepressant treatment and risks for attempts and completions.

In Chapter 6, "Psychotic Features in Major Depressive and Manic Episodes," Coryell reviews the CDS data that have addressed the implications of a diagnosis of schizoaffective disorder and its subtypes, as well as the boundaries between psychotic mood disorders and schizophrenia. This chapter also summarizes the prognostic importance of psychotic features to both manic and depressive episodes.

In Chapter 7, "Development of Mania or Hypomania in the Course of Unipolar Major Depression," Fiedorowicz et al. address a specific issue related to the long-term course of unipolar major depression. Some individuals with unipolar major depression develop hypomania or mania, warranting a change in diagnosis to bipolar disorder. The chapter highlights CDS studies reporting on the incidence of progression to bipolar disorder and determinants thereof. It also reports on the subsequent course of those participants whose first manic or hypomanic episode occurred during prospective follow-up.

The contribution of the CDS to research exploring the comorbidity of substance use and affective disorders is highlighted in Chapter 8, "Comorbidity of Affective and Substance Use Disorders." It was one of the first studies used to examine the prospective course (including predictors of remission and relapse) of alcoholism and major depression in psychiatric patients presenting primarily for treatment. Although the effect of these studies on the future of comorbidity research is evident through their citations, the most direct influence was a National Institute on Drug Abuse–funded prospective study, the Clinfol study, of which many of the improved measures and methods used grew from lessons learned during the CDS. With the upcoming DSM-5, the RDC used in the CDS also warrant mention because the diagnostic approach for substance use disorders is more similar to that used in DSM-5 than any other widely used nomenclature.

In Chapter 9, "Treatment Effectiveness and Safety in the Longitudinal Course of Mood Disorders," Fiedorowicz reviews CDS studies investigating the effectiveness and safety of somatic treatments for mood disorders. Many of these studies were able to use the long-term data of the CDS to answer questions about treatment that could not feasibly be addressed or had not yet been addressed with clinical trial data.

The CDS made many contributions to understanding the relation between personality and depression. The contributions of the CDS are explored further in Chapter 10, "Personality and Mood Disorders." Many of the then-existing theories about personality predisposition to depression were not strongly supported by CDS research. However, increased neuroticism and decreased emotional strength tended to predict subsequent first episodes of depression.

In Chapter 11, "Family History and Genetic Studies in Mood Disorders," Rice reviews findings from analyses of diagnoses in relatives. Early in the course of the CDS, we compared diagnoses made with direct interview with those that used the family history. These procedures were later adapted for the large-scale genetic studies begun in the 1990s. The most striking finding from analysis of the cohort of relatives was the detection of a strong secular trend for MDD, with more recently born individuals having an increased risk. Family analysis showed that schizoaffective disorder, manic subtype, appeared to segregate with bipolar I disorder, whereas the depressed subtype did not. Rice also describes results from a second blind reassessment of all relatives 6 years after their initial assessment.

The CDS was the first study to observe the longitudinal course of unipolar major depression prospectively using a clear and consistent methodology and specific diagnostic criteria. In Chapter 12, "Clinical Course and Outcome of Unipolar Major Depression," Keller and colleagues review the information garnered from the 30 years of study on time to recovery, time to recurrence, and predictors thereof and describe how this information has helped to answer some of the most fundamental questions about MDD, including how to approach patients at different points in their illness, patients with comorbid dysthymia, and patients with substantial social and/or occupational dysfunction.

The CDS also prospectively observed many occurrences of, and recoveries from, bipolar disorder. As Coryell describes in Chapter 13, "Predictors of Course and Outcome of Bipolar Disorder," this study provided the means to describe both typical phase lengths and the risk factors for these changes. The calculation of symptom morbidity in the form of numbers of weeks ill allowed the identification of certain baseline features that had markedly sustained prognostic importance.

In Chapter 14, "Undertreatment of Major Depression," Boland et al. note that although the CDS was not designed to investigate treatment, it offered an opportunity to closely observe the treatment of depression in a natural setting. The conclusions from these observations, first reported in 1982, were surprising: they found that only about one-third of patients who entered the study with MDD received antidepressant medications for an adequate time, and fewer received an adequate dose. These initial reports were met with some skepticism; however, subsequent prospective reports from the CDS and other studies have confirmed these findings. In response to these concerns, the National Depressive and Manic Depressive Association organized a consensus conference on the undertreatment of depression in 1996, which examined the costs of undertreatment to society and suggested some strategies to improve the assessment and treatment of depression. Despite considerable advances and educational efforts subsequent to this conference, the problem of undertreating depression remains a stubborn one. It remains, however, a resolvable one, and Boland and colleagues discuss the clinical implications and future directions needed to help address the gap between knowledge and practice.

In Chapter 15, "Impact of Anxiety Severity on Mood Disorders," Fawcett et al. explore how the CDS used SADS-C (Change Version) ratings that allowed for the measurement of both the presence and the severity of anxiety symptoms in probands with major affective disorders. This led to findings of a significant presence of anxiety symptoms and significant severity levels that were equal in frequency in both unipolar and bipolar disorders. They also found that the severity of anxiety symptoms was associated with poor outcomes over 20 years of follow-up. In addition, severe anxiety symptoms, as well as comorbid panic attacks, were significantly correlated with suicide from weeks up to 1 year of follow-up. Subsequent findings from studies reviewed in this chapter have confirmed these outcomes. This has led to the addition of an anxiety severity rating across mood disorder diagnoses in DSM-5.

In Chapter 16, Fawcett summarizes some key contributions of the CDS to DSM-5, including the spectrum view of mood disorders and the comorbidity of severe anxiety with these disorders.

Summary of the Effect of the Collaborative Depression Study

The CDS's 31 years of longitudinal follow-up lasted far longer than originally planned, largely because the data have proved so informative. The CDS is one of the longest follow-up studies ever done in psychiatry; certainly, it is the most intensive. Data collection has now ended, and 285 empirical reports have been published (as of September 2012). This volume provides a summary of our key findings—findings that have led to a reformulation of the nomenclature of mood disorders and a new understanding of their long-term course, including risk factors for chronicity and recurrence. We wish to thank our participants and their families for staying with us all these years and for providing all the extraordinarily informative data on themselves.

References

Achor RWP, Hazison N, Gifford RW: Hypertension treated with Rauwolfia serpentina (whole root) and with reserpine. JAMA 159:841–845, 1955

Aghajanian GK, Foote WE, Sheard MH: Lysergic acid diethylamide: sensitive neuronal units in the midbrain raphe. Science 161:706–708, 1968

Aghajanian GK, Foote WE, Sheard MH: Action of psychotogenic drugs on single midbrain raphe neurons. J Pharmacol Exp Ther 171:178–187, 1970

American Psychiatric Association: Diagnostic and Statistical Manual of Mental Disorders, 3rd Edition. Washington, DC, American Psychiatric Association, 1980

Blazer D, Swartz M, Woodbury M, et al: Depressive symptoms and depressive diagnoses in a community population: use of a new procedure for analysis of psychiatric classification. Arch Gen Psychiatry 45:1078–1084, 1988

Blazer D, Kessler R, McGonagle K, et al: The prevalence and distribution of major depression in a national community sample: the National Comorbidity Survey. Am J Psychiatry 151:979–986, 1994

Bunney WE, Davis JM: Norepinephrine in depressive reactions. Arch Gen Psychiatry 13:483–494, 1965

Carlsson A, Lindqvist M, Magnusson T: 3,4-Dihydroxyphenlaline and 5-hydroxytryptophan as reserpine antagonists. Nature 180:1200, 1957

Cassano GB, Michelini S, Shear MK, et al: The panic-agoraphobic spectrum: a descriptive approach to the assessment and treatment of subtle symptoms. Am J Psychiatry 154 (6 suppl):27–38, 1997

Chodoff P: The depressive personality: a critical review. Int J Psychiatry 11:196–217, 1973

Clayton PJ: The comorbidity factor: establishing the primary diagnosis in patients with mixed symptoms of anxiety and depression. J Clin Psychiatry 51(suppl):35–39, 1990

Eaton WW, Regier DA, Locke BZ, et al: The Epidemiologic Catchment Area Program of the National Institute of Mental Health. Public Health Rep 96:319–325, 1981

Endicott J, Spitzer RL: A diagnostic interview: the Schedule for Affective Disorders and Schizophrenia. Arch Gen Psychiatry 35:837–844, 1978

Endicott J, Spitzer RL: Use of the Research Diagnostic Criteria and the Schedule for Affective Disorders and Schizophrenia to study affective disorders. Am J Psychiatry 136:52–56, 1979

Feighner JP, Robins E, Guze SB, et al: Diagnostic criteria for use in psychiatric research. Arch Gen Psychiatry 26:57–63, 1972

Gaddum JH: Chemical transmission in the central nervous system. Nature 197:741–743, 1963

Goodwin FK, Murphy DL, Brodie HK, et al: L-DOPA, catecholamines, and behavior: a clinical and biochemical study in depressed patients. Biol Psychiatry 2:341–366, 1970

Haigler HJ, Aghajanian GK: Mescaline and LSD: direct and indirect effects on serotonin-containing neurons in brain. Eur J Pharmacol 21:53–60, 1973

Harris TH: Depression induced by Rauwolfia compounds. Am J Psychiatry 113:950, 1957

Herting C, Axelrod J, Whitby LC: Effect of drugs on the uptake and metabolism of H3-norepinephrine. J Pharmacol Exp Ther 134:146–153, 1961

Hirschfeld RM: History and evolution of the monoamine hypothesis of depression. J Clin Psychiatry 61(suppl 6):4–6, 2000

Hirschfeld RM, Klerman GL, Gough HG, et al: A measure of interpersonal dependency. J Pers Assess 41:610–618, 1977a

Hirschfeld RM, Klerman GL, Schless AP, et al: Modified Life Events of Psychiatric Epidemiology Research Interview (PERI-M). Rockville, MD, National Institute of Mental Health Clinical Research Branch, 1977b

Judd LL, Akiskal HS: The prevalence and disability of bipolar spectrum disorders in the US population: reanalysis of the ECA database taking into account subthreshold cases. J Affect Disord 73(1–2):123–131, 2003

Katz MM, Secunda SK, Hirschfeld RM, et al: NIMH Clinical Research Branch Collaborative Program on the Psychobiology of Depression. Arch Gen Psychiatry 36:765–771, 1979

Keller MB, Lavori PW, Friedman B, et al: The Longitudinal Interval Follow-up Evaluation: a comprehensive method for assessing outcome in prospective longitudinal studies. Arch Gen Psychiatry 44:540–548, 1987

Kessler RC, Nelson CB, McGonagle KA, et al: Comorbidity of DSM-III-R major depressive disorder in the general population: results from the US National Comorbidity Survey. Br J Psychiatry Suppl (30):17–30, 1996

Maas JW, Koslow SH, Davis JM, et al: Biological component of the NIMH Clinical Research Branch Collaborative Program on the Psychobiology of Depression, I: background and theoretical considerations. Psychol Med 10:759–776, 1980

Maser JD, Akiskal HS: Spectrum concepts in major mental disorders. Psychiatr Clin North Am 25:xi–xiii, 2002

Maser JD, Gallup GG Jr, Hicks LE: Tonic immobility in chickens: possible involvement of monoamines. J Comp Physiol Psychol 89:319–328, 1975

Muller JC, Pryer WW, Gibbons JE, et al: Depression and anxiety occurring during Rauwolfia therapy. JAMA 159:836–839, 1955

Regier DA, Goldberg ID, Taube CA: The de facto US mental health services system. Arch Gen Psychiatry 35:685–693, 1978

Schildkraut JJ: The catecholamine hypothesis of affective disorders: a review of supporting evidence. Am J Psychiatry 122:509–521, 1965

Shore PA, Silver SL, Brodie BB: Interaction of reserpine, serotonin, and lysergic acid diethylamide in brain. Science 122:284–285, 1955

Spitzer RL, Endicott J, Robins E: Research Diagnostic Criteria: rationale and reliability. Arch Gen Psychiatry 35:773–782, 1978

Strom-Olsen R, Weil-Malherbe H: Humoral changes in manic-depressive psychosis with particular reference to the excretion of catechol amines in urine. J Ment Sci 104:696–704, 1958

Woolley DW, Shaw E: A biochemical and pharmacological suggestion about certain mental disorders. Science 119:587–588, 1954

World Health Organization: Global Burden of Disease: update 2004. Available at: http://www.who.int/healthinfo/global_burden_disease/GBD_report_2004update_full.pdf. Accessed January 2013.

Zinbarg RE, Barlow DH, Liebowitz M, et al: The DSM-IV field trial for mixed anxiety-depression. Am J Psychiatry 151:1153–1162, 1994

CHAPTER 2

Collaborative Depression Study Procedures and Study Design

Jean Endicott, Ph.D.

THIS CHAPTER CONTAINS brief descriptions of the primary assessment procedures developed or selected for use in those aspects of the Collaborative Depression Study (CDS) discussed in other chapters in this book. Although many additional procedures were used in the CDS, they are not described in this chapter because data collected with them are not discussed in the other chapters. The specific use of the procedures in the CDS is described in the section "Overview of Study Design" later in this chapter. Similarly, the overview of the study design is limited to aspects that are relevant to the other chapters in this volume.

Development of Integrated Collaborative Depression Study Procedures

As noted in Chapter 1 ("Introduction"), the Clinical Studies Committee (CSC) recognized that none of the many different ways of classifying the affective disorders or procedures for collection of diagnostic data had adequate coverage to address the range of issues to be explored in the CDS. The initial focus of the CSC was on the development of new assessment procedures for descriptive psychopathology and alternative ways of making diagnoses suitable for study not only of index subjects but also of their family members and community control subjects. In addition, the CSC wanted to provide a comprehensive description of the multiple aspects of the affective disorders to better test alternative nosological groupings; assess possible prognostic, family, and genetic factors; and evaluate the clinical course and symptom manifestations of affective disorders. To help achieve these aims, the CSC developed and tested a group of integrated procedures: the Research Diagnostic Criteria (RDC), various versions of the Schedule for Affective Disorders and Schizophrenia (SADS), the Family History Research Diagnostic Criteria (FH-RDC), the Longitudinal Interval Follow-Up Evaluation (LIFE), the New Episode/New Condition Report (NE/NCR), and the Suicide Attempt and/or Death Report (GRIM). All of these procedures require good clinical skills and a thorough knowledge of the RDC.

Research Diagnostic Criteria

The first task was to develop a procedure to enable investigators to select relatively homogeneous groups of subjects who met specified criteria for current and lifetime diagnoses. Initial work focused on modification and elaboration of some of the diagnostic criteria developed at the Washington University School of Medicine in St. Louis, Missouri, often referred to as the *Feighner criteria* (Feighner et al. 1972). Many additional sets of diagnostic criteria were added to aid in the differential diagnosis of subtypes of current and lifetime affective disorders and to assess current and lifetime comorbidity of other mental disorders.

The rationales for the specific diagnostic concepts included in the RDC are described in detail elsewhere (Spitzer et al. 1978). Many of the 26 major RDC diagnostic categories (Table 2–1) are further subdivided into non–mutually exclusive subtypes. Major depressive episodes, for example, may be categorized as primary or secondary, recurrent unipolar, psychotic, incapacitating, endogenous, agitated, retarded, situational, or simple and by predominant mood. The joint interview and test-retest κ coefficients of agreement for the major diagnostic categories for both current and lifetime diagnoses indicated high reliability (Andreasen et al. 1981; Keller et al. 1981a, 1981b; Spitzer et al. 1978).

Schedule for Affective Disorders and Schizophrenia

Procedures also were developed to help reduce information variance by standardizing the collection and summarization of clinical information needed to address

TABLE 2–1. Research Diagnostic Criteria diagnoses

Schizophrenia

Schizoaffective disorder–manic

Schizoaffective disorder–depressed

Depressive syndrome superimposed on residual schizophrenia

Manic disorder

Hypomanic disorder

Bipolar with mania (bipolar I)[a]

Bipolar with hypomania (bipolar II)[a]

Major depressive disorder

Minor depressive disorder

Intermittent depressive disorder

Panic disorder

Generalized anxiety disorder

Cyclothymic personality[a]

Labile personality[a]

Briquet's disorder (somatization disorder)[a]

Antisocial personality[a]

Alcoholism

Drug use disorder

Obsessive-compulsive disorder

Phobic disorder

Unspecified functional psychosis

Other psychiatric disorder

Schizotypal features[a]

Currently not mentally ill

Never mentally ill[a]

[a]These conditions are diagnosed on a longitudinal or lifetime basis. All others are diagnosed on the basis of current or past episodes of psychopathology.

the various issues of the CDS. The SADS has three versions—the "regular" version (SADS), the Lifetime version (SADS-L), and the version for measuring change (SADS-C), all described in greater detail elsewhere (Endicott and Spitzer 1978). Each version includes a structured interview guide and items designed specifically for eliciting information relevant to RDC diagnostic categories, to prognosis, and to descriptions of clinical phenomenology. Ratings of the scaled items for all versions of the SADS are made using clearly defined levels of severity for each item, and the interviewer is instructed to use all sources of information and as many general or specific questions as necessary to determine these ratings.

The SADS has two parts. Part I is used to describe features of the current episode of illness with a focus on the time when the symptoms were at their most severe. The coverage is adequate for the interviewer to be able to address differential diagnostic issues and make current RDC diagnoses. Part II describes aspects of psychopathology, functioning, and treatment manifested prior to the current episode and characterizes previous RDC diagnoses (e.g., age at first episode, number of episodes, key clinical features). Selected clinical features that were not specific for a period of illness are also assessed (e.g., social functioning, suicidal behavior). The individual items are grouped in a summary scoring system for various dimensions of psychopathology that have been shown to have high joint and test-retest reliability (e.g., suicidal ideation and behavior, anxiety, manic syndrome) (Endicott and Spitzer 1978).

The SADS-L has the same coverage as Part II of the SADS except that the time period is not limited to the past and includes any current disturbance, if present. The SADS-L was developed to aid in the evaluation of nonpatients such as family members or community subjects. The SADS-L also can be used to cover specified "interval" periods depending on the design of follow-up studies (e.g., since some specific time or event). The reliability of lifetime diagnoses and of individual SADS-L items was assessed with relatives of CDS index subjects (Andreasen et al. 1981), and both short-interval and long-interval test-retest reliabilities for diagnoses and symptoms were found to be quite high.

The SADS-C was developed to aid in evaluation of changes in severity of selected symptoms evaluated at intake and at later times. The items on the SADS-C are included as part of the SADS and in a "stand-alone" procedure. The SADS-C items have the same content as a subset of the scaled items that are contained in Part I of the SADS. However, the SADS-C items are judged for the level of severity during the week preceding the evaluation.

The individual SADS-C items can be grouped into summary scales descriptive of specific dimensions of psychopathology (e.g., depressive mood and ideation). The item selection is such that they can also be scored to provide an extracted Hamilton Depression Rating Scale score (Endicott et al. 1981). The SADS-C summary scales also have been shown to have high internal consistency and high joint interview and test-retest coefficients of reliability (Endicott and Spitzer 1978).

Family History Research Diagnostic Criteria

The FH-RDC include a suggested interview guide and diagnostic criteria for making 14 lifetime family history diagnoses for each relative of interest:

schizophrenia; schizoaffective disorder, manic; schizoaffective disorder, depressed; depression; mania; organic brain syndrome; unspecified functional psychosis; alcoholism; drug use disorder; antisocial personality; other psychiatric disorder; bipolar disorder; recurrent unipolar disorder; and never mentally ill. In addition, data are obtained for any history of suicide attempts, social incapacitation, hospitalization, and treatments for mental disorders. The FH-RDC are somewhat less stringent than the RDC because information obtained indirectly or secondhand is by nature less complete. Andreasen et al. (1977) described the development of the FH-RDC and documented evidence of their reliability.

Longitudinal Interval Follow-Up Evaluation

The LIFE was designed to assess the prospective longitudinal course of psychiatric disorders (Keller et al. 1987). It consists of a semistructured interview guide used to collect detailed psychosocial, psychopathological, and somatic treatment information for 6-month follow-up intervals. The Streamlined Longitudinal Interval Continuation Evaluation (SLICE) is a much reduced version of the LIFE covering follow-up intervals of 1 year. In both, information from subject interviews, family informants, and medical records is used to derive weekly psychiatric status ratings (PSRs), which are ordinal symptom-based scales with categories defined to match the levels of symptoms described in the RDC. The status ratings provide a separate record of the course of each disorder that was initially diagnosed at intake or that developed during the follow-up period. Both record psychosocial and treatment information and link these data temporally to the PSRs. Ratings of videotaped interviews showed excellent reliability and validity for week-by-week PSRs of the major episodic affective disorders, for the timing of changes, and for the summaries of illness course (Keller et al. 1987). The psychosocial items also had generally high reliability and validity.

The LIFE and SLICE use patient and informant reports as well as medical records to describe weekly somatic treatment throughout the follow-up period (e.g., average weekly doses for individual psychotropic drugs, number and frequency of treatments for electroconvulsive therapy). Data from these treatment records yield composite treatment levels for antidepressant, antimanic, antipsychotic, and other summary treatment scores. The LIFE and SLICE were not designed to collect systematic data on psychotherapeutic treatments, and, therefore, the effect of psychotherapeutic intervention is unknown for the CDS subjects, a limitation that we state in publications.

The LIFE and SLICE assess the level of functioning for the following psychosocial areas: 1) work, 2) household duties (rated for both males and females), 3) school, 4) interpersonal relationships with both family and friends,

5) recreation, 6) life satisfaction as an assessment of the subject's level of contentment with various areas of his or her life, and 7) global social adjustment. An overall composite measure of psychosocial functioning, the Range of Impaired Functioning Tool (LIFE-RIFT), combines several of the individual functioning scores. The development and testing of the LIFE-RIFT are described in detail by Leon et al. (1999).

New Episode/New Condition Report

The NE/NCR, developed by Keller and Shapiro (1978a), records details of all new episodes of disorders manifested during the follow-up period being covered. It contains 1) a summary of treatment status and suicidal behavior during the new episode or condition, 2) symptom checklists for depressive and manic or hypomanic syndromes, 3) an RDC diagnostic classification of the new episode or condition, and 4) the Global Assessment Scale ratings for the severity of the episode or condition at its worst.

Suicide Attempt and/or Death Report (GRIM)

The GRIM, also developed by Keller and Shapiro (1978b), describes suicidal behavior and cause of death and details of the circumstances surrounding the event (e.g., intoxication, recent life events, presence of delusions or hallucinations). For nonlethal attempts, the suicidal intent and medical threat to life are rated on a 6-point severity scale. Information on subject suicide attempts or completions or death from other causes is obtained from relatives and treating professionals, from medical records obtained by the center, or from the National Death Index.

Personality Measures

The CSC also recognized the importance of personality features to the study of subjects with major affective disorders and their relatives. Initially, a 436-item self-report personality battery was derived by selecting 17 scales from the following instruments: General Activity, Restraint, Ascendance, Sociability, Emotional Stability, Objectivity, and Thoughtfulness from the Guilford-Zimmerman Temperament Survey (Guilford and Zimmerman 1949); Emotional Reliance on Another Person, Lack of Social Self-Confidence, and Assertion of Autonomy from the Interpersonal Dependency Inventory (Hirschfeld et al. 1977); Orality, Obsessionality, and Hysterical Pattern from the short form of the Lazare-Klerman-Armor Personality Inventory (Lazare et al. 1966); Neuroticism and Extraversion from the Maudsley Personality Inventory (Eysenck 1962); and Ego Resiliency and Ego Control from the Minnesota Multiphasic Personality Inventory (MMPI; Hathaway and McKinley 1951). The General Behavior Inventory (Dupue et al. 1981) was added to the battery later to assess dysthymic and cyclothymic tendencies. With the exception of the two scales from the MMPI, the subjects were instructed to answer questions according to their "usual self" (i.e., their typical way of acting or feeling). Hirschfeld et al. (1983) described the rationale behind the need for a composite battery, the selection of the specific measures, and the modified instructions. Key findings based on CDS personality assessments are presented in Chapter 10 ("Personality and Mood Disorders") of this volume.

Overview of Study Design

As noted previously, in this section, I focus on those aspects of the study design that are most relevant for having a better understanding of the chapters that follow, summarizing key findings from the CDS.

Training and Monitoring of Clinical Raters

Each site selected raters who had some clinical experience with subjects with mental disorders, and all raters underwent intensive training in use of the RDC, SADS, FH-RDC, and LIFE. Videotapes, case vignettes, and joint interview/rating sessions were used in the training (Gibbon et al. 1981). Within-site and cross-site reliability were assessed (Andreasen et al. 1981, 1982; Keller et al. 1981a, 1981b, 1983). The raters and site protocol monitors had regularly scheduled conference calls and meetings to guard against rater drift over time and to address diagnostic issues. Senior diagnosticians at the New York site were available for consultation and, as noted later in this chapter, reviewed all intake diagnostic evaluations.

Selection of Index Subjects

Index subjects were selected during the period from 1978 to 1981. Potential subjects were screened at the five centers to determine whether they met criteria for a current depressive or manic syndrome; were Caucasian (to test genetic hypotheses); spoke English; were 17 years or older; had no evidence of an organic mental disorder, mental deficiency, or terminal illness; lived in the area; and had knowledge of their biological parents. In an effort to fill preassigned diagnostic cell sizes, subjects were then further screened and recruited if they met RDC for one of the five following lifetime disorders: schizoaffective ($n=80$), bipolar I ($n=163$), bipolar II ($n=114$), major depressive disorder ($n=598$), or chronic minor or intermittent depressive disorders ($n=6$). The chronic minor or intermittent depressive disorders group was later dropped because of limited recruitment. A sample of 955 index subjects was selected, including 171 from Boston, Massachusetts, 172 from Chicago, Illinois, 246 from Iowa City, Iowa, 117 from New York, and 249 from St. Louis, Missouri. The index subjects had considerable heterogeneity with regard to lifetime co-morbid mental disorders (e.g., alcoholism, $n = 283$; drug abuse, $n = 133$; panic disorder, $n = 41$; generalized anxiety disorder, $n = 57$; and phobic disorder, $n = 59$). Chronic minor or intermittent depressive disorder also was present before the onset of the index affective episode in 153 of the subjects. The mean age at intake was 38 years (range = 17–79), 58% were women, and 80% were inpatients. Although the intake procedures did not result in a sample representative of all people with affective disorders, the CDS sample does represent individuals with moderate to severe illness. Inclusion of subjects with comorbid nonaffective disorders may render the CDS data more generalizable to clinical practice than do studies with more restrictive inclusion criteria.

Index Subject Intake Evaluations

The SADS and RDC were completed at intake by using all sources of information, and a narrative was written to justify the ratings and diagnoses. This information was updated at discharge (inpatients) or 2 months after intake (outpatients). All SADS ratings, RDC diagnoses, and the narratives were reviewed by senior clinicians both at the originating data collection center and at the New York center. Additional intake data were collected via self-report symptom measures; family reports of symptoms; detailed demographic questions; an intelligence test; self-reported current and past medical history; and assessments of recent life stresses, personality, and current personal resources.

Index Subject Follow-Up Evaluations

Follow-up evaluations began immediately after intake and were summarized with the LIFE every 6 months up to 60 months and yearly thereafter with the SLICE. Raters completed NE/NCRs or GRIMs for the period under study if their use was warranted. Lifetime RDC diagnoses were updated at years 5, 10, 15, 20, and 25 or at the time of leaving the study, and information on reasons for any change in lifetime diagnoses were noted. The personality measures were completed again at 1 and 5 years, and demographic information was updated at the 5-, 20-, and 25-year evaluations.

Evaluations of First-Degree Relatives

Raters used the FH-RDC to collect diagnostic data for all first-degree relatives of all index subjects. When possible, they interviewed two informants, the index subject and one other "best" family informant, and produced a "consensus" FH-RDC diagnosis. When conflicting information occurred, the most positive diagnosis was usually given. The "family history" sample consisted of 4,373 first-degree relatives who were at least 17 years old. The "family study" sample consisted of 2,216 first-degree relatives of the 609 index subjects included in the family study. All of these relatives were interviewed directly with the SADS-L. A consensus pedigree for each index subject included in the family study showed all consensus FH-RDC diagnoses, the SADS-L diagnoses, and "clinical consensus" diagnoses that took into account all sources of information. Six years after the initial family study evaluation, an effort was made to contact and reevaluate those family study relatives as well as any relatives who had come of age or who had refused the initial SADS-L interview, resulting in 2,043 sixth-year diagnostic evaluations. Raters also assessed psychosocial variables, life stresses, and personal resources and obtained personality batteries for the family study relatives at both the initial and the 6-year evaluations.

Evaluation of Other Study Samples

The CDS included various smaller groups of subjects selected for comparison with subsets of index subjects or first-degree relatives. Diagnostic (SADS-L/RDC) and psychosocial assessments were made for 108 psychosocial control subjects and 469 family study control subjects, as well as 360 spouses of index subjects.

Clinical Implications

- Clinical raters with various experience and training can be trained to achieve and maintain high within- and cross-site joint and test-retest agreement of both clinical ratings and diagnosis of current and lifetime conditions.
- Index subjects, their relatives, and community control subjects can be recruited and will continue participation in long-term follow-up evaluations yielding detailed information that cannot be obtained in cross-sectional evaluations.
- Continued use of the same study procedures in a long-term prospective project allows the analysis of changes over time, with a focus not only on diagnoses but also on factors such as the effects of aging, changes in treatment, and other issues that require evaluation of repeated episodes.

References

Andreasen NC, Endicott J, Spitzer RL, et al: The family history method using diagnostic criteria: reliability and validity. Arch Gen Psychiatry 34:1229–1235, 1977

Andreasen NC, Grove WM, Shapiro RW, et al: Reliability of lifetime diagnosis: a multicenter collaborative perspective. Arch Gen Psychiatry 38:400–405, 1981

Andreasen NC, McDonald-Scott P, Grove WM, et al: Assessment of reliability in multicenter collaborative research with a videotape approach. Am J Psychiatry 139:876–882, 1982

Dupue RA, Slater JF, Wolfstetter-Kausch H, et al: A behavioral paradigm for identifying persons at risk for bipolar depressive disorder: a conceptual framework and five validation studies. J Abnorm Psychol 90:381–437, 1981

Endicott J, Spitzer RL: A diagnostic interview: the Schedule for Affective Disorders and Schizophrenia. Arch Gen Psychiatry 35:837–844, 1978

Endicott J, Cohen J, Nee J, et al: Hamilton Depression Rating Scale extracted from regular and change versions of the Schedule for Affective Disorders and Schizophrenia. Arch Gen Psychiatry 38:98–103, 1981

Eysenck HJ: The Maudsley Personality Inventory. San Diego, CA, Educational and Industrial Testing Service, 1962

Feighner JP, Robins E, Guze SB, et al: Diagnostic criteria for use in psychiatric research. Arch Gen Psychiatry 26:57–63, 1972

Gibbon M, McDonald-Scott P, Endicott J: Mastering the art of research interviewing: a model training procedure for diagnostic evaluation. Arch Gen Psychiatry 38:1259–1262, 1981

Guilford JP, Zimmerman WS: The Guilford-Zimmerman Temperament Survey Manual. Beverly Hills, CA, Sheridan Supply, 1949

Hathaway SR, McKinley JC: The Minnesota Multiphasic Personality Inventory, Revised. New York, Psychological Corporation, 1951

Hirschfeld RM, Klerman GL, Gough HG, et al: A measure of interpersonal dependency. J Pers Assess 41:610–618, 1977

Hirschfeld RMA, Klerman GL, Clayton PJ, et al: Effects of the depressive state on trait measurement. Am J Psychiatry 140:695–699, 1983

Keller MB, Shapiro RW: New Episode/New Condition Report (NE/NCR). Boston, MA, Massachusetts General Hospital, 1978

Keller MB, Shapiro RW: Suicide Attempt and/or Death Report (GRIM). Boston, MA, Massachusetts General Hospital, 1978

Keller MB, Lavori PW, Andreasen NC, et al: Test-retest reliability of assessing psychiatrically ill patients in a multi-center design. J Psychiatr Res 16:213–227, 1981a

Keller MB, Lavori PW, McDonald-Scott P, et al: Reliability of lifetime diagnoses and symptoms in patients with a current psychiatric disorder. J Psychiatr Res 16:229–240, 1981b

Keller MB, Lavori PW, McDonald-Scott P, et al: The reliability of retrospective treatment reports. Psychiatry Res 9:81–88, 1983

Keller MB, Lavori PW, Friedman B, et al: The longitudinal interval follow-up evaluation: a comprehensive method for assessing outcome in prospective longitudinal studies. Arch Gen Psychiatry 44:540–548, 1987

Lazare A, Klerman GL, Arthor DJ: Oral, obsessive, and hysterical personality patterns: an investigation of psychoanalytic concepts by means of factor analysis. Arch Gen Psychiatry 14:624–630, 1966

Leon AC, Solomon DA, Mueller TI, et al: The Range of Impaired Functioning Tool (LIFE-RIFT): a brief measure of functional impairment. Psychol Med 29:869–878, 1999

Spitzer RL, Endicott J, Robins E: Research Diagnostic Criteria: rationale and reliability. Arch Gen Psychiatry 35:773–782, 1978

CHAPTER 3

Dimensional Symptomatic Structure of the Long-Term Course of Unipolar Major Depressive Disorder

Lewis L. Judd, M.D.

Pamela J. Schettler, Ph.D.

Hagop S. Akiskal, M.D.

Martin B. Keller, M.D.

BEGINNING IN THE LATE 1990S, the Collaborative Depression Study (CDS) research group at the University of California at San Diego (Lewis L. Judd, M.D., Hagop S. Akiskal, M.D., Pamela J. Schettler, Ph.D., and Jack D. Maser, Ph.D.) introduced a dimensional paradigm for description and analysis of the long-term, naturalistic course of unipolar major depressive disorder (MDD). Because of their clinical expertise and prior research (Akiskal et al. 1997; Judd 1997; Judd et al. 1996, 1997a, 1997b), these investigators believed that the prevailing focus on major depressive episodes (MDEs), although very important, would be more complete if it included a description of less severe depressive symptom states that occur during the long-term course of MDD. They embarked on a series of studies (Judd et al. 1998a, 1998b, 2000a, 2000b) that used data from the National Institute of Mental Health (NIMH) CDS (Katz and Klerman 1979; Katz et al. 1979).

CDS data provide a unique resource for examining all levels of depressive severity in the long-term course of MDD. Weekly psychiatric status ratings (PSRs), captured with variants of the Longitudinal Interval Follow-Up Evaluation (LIFE) interviews (Keller et al. 1987) as described in Chapter 2 ("Collaborative Depression Study Procedures and Study Design") of this volume, are used to record symptom severity on every Research Diagnostic Criteria (RDC) condition (Spitzer et al. 1977) present in CDS patients by that point during follow-up. PSRs, which are anchored to diagnostic thresholds for RDC disorders, allow depressive symptom severity for each week of follow-up to be assigned to one of four categories: 1) meeting the diagnostic threshold for MDD, 2) being less severe but meeting the diagnostic threshold for minor depression or dysthymia, 3) being present at a subsyndromal depressive level below the threshold for minor depression or dysthymia, or 4) being entirely absent (asymptomatic).

Early analyses (Keller et al. 1992) showed that CDS patients spend a median of only 32% of weeks from the start to the end of an MDE at the full syndromal level of severity; the remainder (majority) of time in the episode is spent with minor or subsyndromal depressive symptoms. At the other end of the severity spectrum, the consensual definition of MDE recovery was a period of 8 or more consecutive weeks with no more than minimal symptoms of the MDE. Clinical experience suggested that the presence of minimal symptoms during resolution of an MDE reflects an ongoing, active state of the illness rather than a "recovered" or truly intermorbid state and that true MDE recovery occurs only when all symptoms of the episode are removed.

Findings based on *all* levels of symptomatic activity during the long-term course of MDD, summarized in the remainder of this chapter, have provided unexpected new information and have established the importance of the dimensional paradigm for clinical research as well as for effective long-term management of this illness. (Findings and implications based on a dimensional analysis of bipolar disorders are presented in Chapter 4, "Dimensional Symptomatic Structure of the Long-Term Course of Bipolar I and Bipolar II Disorders," of this volume.) It should be emphasized that the evidence for the paradigm shift described in this chapter pertains only to patients meeting diagnostic criteria for unipolar MDD, based on a lifetime history of one or more MDEs with no evidence of bipolarity, schizoaffective disorder, or schizophrenia. Also, because MDD patients entering the CDS were seeking treatment at tertiary care centers, they likely had presentations that differed in complexity and severity from those of individuals seen in primary care settings or individuals who were ill and not seeking treatment. Thus, the findings may not generalize to patients with MDD in all clinical settings.

Methods

For a description of major CDS samples and procedures for diagnosis and follow-up, see Chapter 2 of this volume.

Subjects

Analysis of the dimensional symptomatic structure of the long-term course of unipolar MDE was based on systematic follow-up data for CDS patients, assessed at 6-month intervals for the first 5 years, then yearly to a maximum of 31 years after intake. Among the subjects who entered the CDS in a definite MDE by RDC (Spitzer et al. 1977), which are very similar to DSM-IV-TR (American Psychiatric Association 2000) criteria, 424 were selected who had no evidence of bipolar disorder (bipolar I disorder, bipolar II disorder, or cyclothymia), schizoaffective disorder, or schizophrenia—either prior to intake or by the end of follow-up. Because the goal was to describe long-term course, 57 subjects with less than 2 years of follow-up data were omitted. The dimensional structure of the long-term course of unipolar MDD is described for the resulting sample of 367 subjects. Table 3–1 summarizes their demographic and clinical characteristics and length of CDS follow-up (median = 18.4 years). The unique nature of the CDS is evidenced by the fact that nearly half of these subjects (48.2%) were followed up for 20 years or longer.

Depressive Symptom Severity Levels

Weekly depressive symptom severity was rated with the PSR scales for MDD, minor depressive disorder, and intermittent depressive disorder. For the analyses presented here, each follow-up week was assigned to one of four mutually exclusive depressive symptom severity categories as shown in Table 3–2, independent of whether the subject was in an RDC episode at that time. The four categories represent a continuum of levels of illness activity anchored to symptom severity thresholds defining subtypes of depressive episodes or the asymptomatic status:

> *Level 1*—asymptomatic status; return to usual self, with no depressive symptoms
> *Level 2*—mildly severe symptom(s) below the diagnostic threshold for MDD or minor depressive disorder, referred to here as *subsyndromal depressive* symptoms
> *Level 3*—moderately severe symptoms, at the threshold for minor depressive disorder or its long-term variant, dysthymia
> *Level 4*—most severe symptoms, at the diagnostic threshold for MDD

TABLE 3–1. Demographic and clinical characteristics and length of prospective follow-up for 367 Collaborative Depression Study (CDS) patients with unipolar major depressive disorder and at least 2 years of follow-up data

Intake characteristics	Intake unipolar MDE sample
Demographics	
Age (years, mean [SD; range])	40.1 [14.9; 17–79]
Female gender (n [%])	226 [61.6]
Education—some college (n [%])	188 [51.2]
Marital status[a] (n [%])	
Married/living together	195 [53.4]
Separated/widowed/divorced	75 [20.6]
Never married	95 [26.0]
Episode history	
Age at onset of first affective episode (years, mean [SD; range])	29.6 [14.4; 3–72]
Onset of first affective episode before age 21 (n [%])	118 [32.2]
Number of lifetime affective episodes (including intake) (n [%])	
1 (first episode)	107 [29.2]
2 or 3	165 [45.0]
≥4	95 [25.9]
Clinical characteristics	
Inpatient status (n [%])	272 [74.1]
Global Assessment Scale (GAS) for worst period in episode[b] (mean [SD])	38.6 [10.7]
Length of CDS follow-up (years)	
Mean (SD)	17.3 (9.7)
Median	18.4

TABLE 3–1. Demographic and clinical characteristics and length of prospective follow-up for 367 Collaborative Depression Study (CDS) patients with unipolar major depressive disorder and at least 2 years of follow-up data *(continued)*

Intake characteristics	Intake unipolar MDE sample
Range	2–31
2–9 (*n* [%])	111 [30.2]
10–19 (*n* [%])	79 [21.5]
20–29 (*n* [%])	159 [43.3]
30–31 (*n* [%])	18 [4.9]

Note. Patients who entered the CDS in a definite major depressive episode (MDE) and had no lifetime evidence of bipolarity (bipolar I disorder, bipolar II disorder, or cyclothymia), schizoaffective disorder, or schizophrenia by the end of CDS follow-up. Analysis of long-term follow-up course is based on subjects with at least 2 years (104 weeks) of follow-up data rated "fair" or better in terms of accuracy (i.e., excluding weeks deemed to have "poor" or "very poor" data).
[a]Marital status information is missing for two subjects.
[b]GAS score measures severity of symptoms and impairment. Scores range from 1 (most severe and impaired) to 100 (superior functioning with no symptoms). A mean of 38.6 represents major impairment in several areas, or some impairment in reality testing or communication, or at least one suicide attempt.

TABLE 3–2. Classification of depressive symptom severity levels based on weekly psychiatric status ratings (PSRs) across all depressive conditions

Depressive symptom severity level	Major depression (6-point PSR scale)[a]	Minor depression (3-point PSR scale)[b]	DSM-III depressive conditions[c] (3-point PSR scale)[b]
1 Asymptomatic: no depressive symptoms of the episode; return to usual self	1	1	1
2 Subsyndromal level: depressive symptoms below the MinD/dysthymia level	1	1	2 or 3
	1	2	(Any)[d]
	2	1 or 2	(Any)

TABLE 3–2. Classification of depressive symptom severity levels based on weekly psychiatric status ratings (PSRs) across all depressive conditions *(continued)*

Depressive symptom severity level	Major depression (6-point PSR scale)[a]	Minor depression (3-point PSR scale)[b]	DSM-III depressive conditions[c] (3-point PSR scale)[b]
3 Affective symptoms at the MinD/dysthymia level	1	3	(Any)
	2	3	(Any)
	3	(Any)	(Any)
	4	(Any)	(Any)
4 Affective symptoms at the MDD level	5	(Any)	(Any)
	6	(Any)	(Any)

Note.   Read across the table for combinations of PSR values that result in classifying a particular week at a given symptom severity level. For example, a patient would be classified at the minor depression or dysthymia level for the week he or she was rated as PSR 3 or 4 on the 6-point major depression scale or PSR 3 on the 3-point minor depression or dysthymia scale with a PSR 1 or 2 on the 6-point major depression scale. MDD=RDC major depressive disorder; MinD=RDC minor or intermittent depressive or dysthymic disorder.

[a]Six-point weekly PSR scale values: 1=asymptomatic, returned to usual self; 2=residual/mild affective symptoms; 3=partial remission, moderate symptoms or impairment; 4=marked/major symptoms or impairment; 5=meets definite criteria without prominent psychotic symptoms or extreme impairment; 6=meets definite criteria with prominent psychotic symptoms or extreme impairment.

[b]Three-point weekly PSR scale values: 1=asymptomatic, returned to usual self; 2=meets probable criteria (mild symptoms); 3=meets definite criteria (severe symptoms).

[c]Weekly symptom severity level is assigned based on each week's ratings on all depressive conditions, regardless of whether the patient was in a Research Diagnostic Criteria (RDC) episode at that time. Rated affective conditions include RDC major depressive disorder (MDD); RDC minor or intermittent depressive or dysthymic disorder (MinD); and DSM-III (American Psychiatric Association 1980) atypical depression (code 296.82) and adjustment disorder with depressed mood (code 309.00). Weekly symptom severity levels are mutually exclusive.

[d]"(Any)" indicates any PSR value of this affective condition qualifies for the given symptom severity level, in conjunction with the values shown for other depressive conditions. For example, a given week is classified at the MDD level based on a PSR value of 5 or 6 for MDD, regardless of PSR values for any other depressive condition.

Findings

Chronicity of Major Depressive Disorder

Over the past two decades, evidence has emerged from the CDS (Coryell et al. 1990; Keller et al. 1992; Mueller et al. 1999) as well as other research groups (Angst and Preisig 1995; Angst et al. 2003; Brodaty et al. 2001; Hoencamp et al. 2001) indicating that MDD is primarily a chronic, often lifelong illness with powerful tendencies for depressive episodes to reappear quickly after apparent MDD resolution (termed a *relapse*) or for a new episode to appear at a later point in the subject's lifetime (termed a *recurrence*).

Major depressive illness tends to have its onset early in life. The cohort of patients entering the CDS in an MDE had a mean age at affective illness onset of 29.6 (SD=14.4) years. This was slightly later than found for community samples in the Epidemiologic Catchment Area (ECA) study (27.4 years) (Weissman et al. 1988) or National Comorbidity Survey Replication (NCS-R) (26.2 years) (Kessler et al. 2010). Nearly one-third of the CDS sample (32.2%) had experienced their first depressive episode before age 21. Although a substantial portion (29.2%) entered the CDS during their first lifetime depressive episode, one-fourth of the sample (25.9%) had experienced three or more previous episodes. Systematic, prospective follow-up data for CDS subjects show the true picture of MDD chronicity.

In Chapter 12 ("Clinical Course and Outcome of Unipolar Major Depression") of this volume, Keller and colleagues provide a detailed description of the chronicity and high cumulative probability of relapse and recurrence of depressive episodes for patients with MDD—updating and extending previously published reports with analysis of the final CDS database, which includes up to 31 years of follow-up. Findings from the CDS presented in Chapter 12 establish the duration of MDEs and the recovery intervals between them according to the current consensus definition of recovery.

An alternative way of describing chronicity in MDD is the percentage of weeks during the entire course of follow-up that patients entering the CDS were symptomatic from their illness with *any* level of severity of depressive symptoms (i.e., with symptoms at the major, minor/dysthymic, or subsyndromal level of severity). New analysis of the weekly course of MDD during up to 31 years of follow-up (median=18.4 years) showed that patients were symptomatic for most of the follow-up period, experiencing some level of depressive symptoms during a mean of 55.4% (SD=35.2%) of weeks. This finding is in striking contrast to the mean of 41.9% (SD=33.1%) of weeks of follow-up that these MDD subjects spent in a depressive episode (major, minor, or dysthymic) during the same period. Further analysis showed that subjects with MDD experienced subsyndromal depressive symptoms during nearly one-third of the weeks (mean = 31.7%; SD = 36.3%) when they were not in episodes of major or minor/dysthymic depression. Thus, inclusion of subsyndromal depressive symptoms considerably extends the picture of the true chronicity of depressive symptoms in MDD.

In summary, the cumulative scientific evidence indicates that MDD is typically a chronic, relapsing illness with multiple recurrences rather than one involving a single, isolated, acute depressive episode, and that subjects with MDD typically experience some symptoms of their illness during most of their long-term course.

Dimensional Expression of Depressive Symptoms in Major Depressive Disorder

Compelling evidence from the CDS follow-up to 31 years (Figure 3–1) showed that the long-term symptomatic course of MDD is expressed as a dimensional continuum of depressive severity, as follows. Severe symptoms, at the major depressive diagnostic threshold, occur during a mean of 14.8% (SD = 19.9%) of the weeks during the long-term course of illness. Moderately severe symptoms, at the diagnostic threshold for minor depression (if less than 2 years) or its chronic variant, dysthymia (if present for 2 years or longer), are present during a mean of 24.2% (SD = 23.0%) of the weeks during follow-up, making this the most common symptomatic severity level during the long-term course of illness. Mild symptoms (i.e., those of subsyndromal, or subthreshold, severity, at a level below that used to diagnose minor depression or dysthymia) occur during a mean of 16.4% (SD = 19.3%) of the follow-up weeks. An additional indication of the dimensional expression of depressive symptoms in MDD comes from the fact that 95.1% of the patients with MDD and 2 or more years of follow-up data experience all four (75.2%) or at least three (19.9%) of these depressive symptom severity levels during the long-term course of their illness.

It is noteworthy that the percentage of time spent at each level of depressive symptom severity or the asymptomatic status, reported here on the basis of up to 31 years of follow-up data per subject, is nearly identical to that published earlier when follow-up data were available for up to 12 years per subject (Judd et al. 1998a). This correspondence suggests striking stability of the symptomatic structure of MDD over subjects' long-term life course. This stability is consistent with a subsequent finding (Coryell et al. 2009) that the percentage of weeks CDS subjects spent in MDEs remained stable across successive decades of their life.

According to the dimensional paradigm, the different levels of depressive symptom severity observed during the course of MDD illness represent stages along a continuum of symptomatic expression. Each level of depressive symptom severity is a different phase of illness intensity and activity but is an integral component of the same illness, namely, MDD.

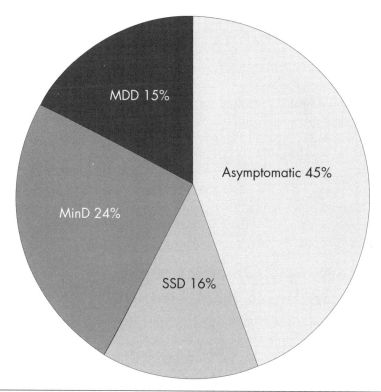

FIGURE 3–1. Mean percentage of weeks in each category of depressive symptom severity during long-term follow-up (median = 18.4 years) of 367 Collaborative Depression Study patients with unipolar major depressive disorder (MDD).

Asymptomatic = no depressive symptoms (usual self); MinD = minor depression/dysthymia threshold; SSD = subsyndromal depressive symptoms (below MinD threshold). *Source.* Reprinted from Judd LL: "Dimensional Paradigm of the Long-Term Course of Unipolar Major Depressive Disorder." *Depression and Anxiety* 29:167–171, 2012. Used with permission.

Longitudinal Prevalence of Minor Depression or Dysthymia and Subsyndromal Depressive Symptoms in Major Depressive Disorder

Early findings from the CDS (Keller et al. 1983a) helped call attention to the phenomenon of MDEs superimposed on episodes of dysthymia (chronic minor depression), a condition known as *double depression,* which affected one in four patients entering the CDS in an acute MDE (see Chapter 12 for further discussion of double depression). In addition, a theoretical perspective has been offered that considers dysthymic traits as one of the underlying structures for major affective illness (Akiskal 1983; Akiskal et al. 1997; Kovacs et al. 1994). This perspective also pertains to patients with a predominantly bipolar course (Akiskal 1994). Thus, it is not surprising that depression at the severity level defining minor depression or dysthymia constitutes the most frequent symptomatic state in the long-term course of MDD. What may be surprising is that on the continuum of depressive severity levels, symptoms at the minor depression or dysthymia level (24.2% of weeks) and subsyndromal depressive symptoms below that level (mean=16.4% of weeks), when taken together (mean=42.3% of weeks), are 2.7 times more common over time than symptoms at the MDE severity threshold (mean=14.8% of weeks).

Even though MDD traditionally has been defined by MDEs, recent evidence shows that most of the long-term symptomatic course of MDD occurs at minor and subthreshold symptom severity levels.

Dynamic Symptomatic Course of Major Depressive Disorder

In earlier reports (Judd 1997; Judd et al. 1994), investigators concluded that the different symptomatic forms of depression commonly seen during the course of MDD were probably discrete depressive disorders or "subtypes" as described by the current official nomenclature in DSM-IV-TR (American Psychiatric Association 2000) and ICD-10 (World Health Organization 1992). Recent evidence of the dynamic course of MDD within a given subject came from secondary analysis of the ECA community subjects who were found to have a surprising degree of depressive symptom fluctuation between their initial diagnostic interview (Wave I) and the identical follow-up interview (Wave II) 1 year later (Judd 1997; Judd et al. 1997a). For example, of the 201 subjects diagnosed with major depression at Wave I, only 28% had symptoms that met diagnostic criteria for major depression at the Wave II interview 1 year later, whereas 23% (apparently all who had double depression at Wave I) had symptoms that met the criteria for dysthymic disorder at Wave II, 15% had a decreased number of depressive symptoms such that they were given the diagnosis of acute minor depression at Wave II, and 13% had reduced symptoms enough to fall into the subsyndromal depressive symptom category. Of the subjects with major depression at Wave I, in only 21% had all of their symptoms abated so that they were asymptomatic 1 year later. A similar degree of depressive symptom fluctuation occurred for subjects in other Wave I depressive symptom or disorder categories.

During the course of up to 30 years of systematic follow-up, individual CDS subjects changed depressive symptom status (between MDD, minor or dysthymic, and subsyndromal depressive symptom severity levels or the asymptomatic status) a mean of 1.5 (SD = 1.3) times per year during all of follow-up. Of the subjects, 23% had more than two depressive symptom status changes per year, averaged across all of follow-up.

These findings provide strong evidence that patients with MDD have a dynamic symptomatic course, alternating among different levels of depressive symptom severity, including the asymptomatic state, as the course of their illness waxes and wanes over time. Prospective longitudinal research with frequent follow-up evaluations is essential for providing a true picture of the dynamic symptomatic course, which cannot be ascertained from acute cross-sectional studies.

Psychosocial Disability Associated With Depressive Symptom Severity Levels in Major Depressive Disorder

Depressive symptoms below the syndromal threshold of MDD often have been ignored and their clinical relevance questioned because it had not been empirically established that minor or subthreshold depressions are associated with significant harmful psychosocial dysfunction—a key criterion proposed to determine when a condition reaches the status of a disorder (Wakefield 1992). One of the earliest studies to show that subsyndromal depressions are associated with psychosocial disability was the large Medical Outcomes Study (Greenfield and Ware 1989). Several secondary analyses of the NIMH ECA data (Judd 1997; Judd et al. 1994, 1997a, 1997b, 2002) compared subjects with subsyndromal depressive symptoms with subjects with no depressive symptoms. Subsyndromal depression was defined as two or more distressing or impairing symptoms of depression present most every day, for most of the day, 2 weeks or more in duration, in subjects whose symptoms did not meet diagnostic criteria for major, minor, or dysthymic depression. Compared with subjects with no depressive symptoms, the subjects with subthreshold depressive symptoms had significantly higher lifetime use of psychiatric inpatient and outpatient services, use of emergency department services, need for public assistance, and history of suicide attempts.

Following up the findings from community-based epidemiological data, the unique resource of the CDS was used to examine psychosocial disability associated with each level of depressive symptom severity *within the same subject* over time (Judd et al. 2000a). Monthly ratings of psychosocial disability were obtained in the CDS for each month of follow-up years 3–5, and the final month of years 6–31, with variations of the LIFE interview form (see Chapter 2 of this volume). Ratings were made for individual domains of everyday life functions (e.g., work/employment, household duties, relationships with spouse or part-ner), as well as a rating of overall (global) psychosocial function. For the 2000 study, monthly psychosocial ratings in follow-up years 3–12 were analyzed for months spent entirely at one of the three levels of depressive symptom severity or the asymptomatic status. Random (mixed) regression analysis was used to model the relation between each impairment rating (dependent variable) and the four depressive symptom categories (independent variable). Mean levels of global psychosocial function (disability or impairment) are graphed in Figure 3–2, which shows a significant progressive stepwise increase in psychosocial impair-ment (decrease in function) with each increment of depressive symptom sever-ity, within the same subjects. When subjects with MDD are asymptomatic, disability is minimal, and psychosocial function normalizes and is rated as "good." When the same subjects experience subsyndromal depressive symp-toms, their psychosocial function is rated between "good" and "fair"; when their symptoms increase to the level of minor depression or dysthymia, psychosocial function is rated between "fair" and "poor"; and when their symptoms reach the threshold of major depression, their disability increases and psychosocial func-tion is rated between "poor" and "very poor." This progression indicates that psychosocial impairment in MDD is state dependent: When the subject is expe-riencing any level of depressive symptoms, even subthreshold symptoms, psy-chosocial function is significantly impaired; however, when symptoms abate and the subject is asymptomatic, function normalizes to "good" levels. It is noteworthy that when compared with control subjects with no current mental disorder, subjects with MDD show a subtle but significantly higher mean level of psychosocial disability during asymptomatic periods. It remains to be deter-mined whether this difference gradually disappears as subjects remain asymp-tomatic for an extended time.

These findings indicate that every level of severity of depressive symp-toms, even those below the threshold for minor depression or dysthymia, is associated with significant impairment, thereby meeting the criterion of harmful dysfunction that defines the presence of a clinically relevant disorder (Wakefield 1992). In addition, the mean level of psychosocial function associ-ated with the MDD threshold (falling between "poor" and "very poor") con-firms the very disabling effect of the severest expression of unipolar depressive illness.

Importance of Asymptomatic Recovery From Major Depressive Episodes

Perhaps the most vexing problem for patients, their families, and clinicians in the management of MDD is the tendency for patients in a MDE to relapse and episodes to recur throughout the course of the unipolar depressive illness. De-

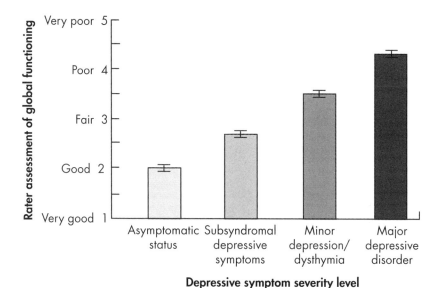

FIGURE 3–2. Mean rating of global psychosocial functioning by depressive symptom severity level during long-term follow-up of Collaborative Depression Study patients with unipolar major depressive disorder.

Based on mixed model repeated measures analysis of functioning during months when the same subject was experiencing different levels of symptom severity. Change in functioning associated with each stepwise change in depressive symptom severity was significant at $P < 0.001$.

Source. Reprinted from Judd LL: "Dimensional Paradigm of the Long-Term Course of Unipolar Major Depressive Disorder." *Depression and Anxiety* 29:167–171, 2012. Used with permission.

spite reports that some specific therapeutic strategies significantly decrease or delay episode relapse, clinically pragmatic strategies for consistently reducing chronicity in recurrent MDD remain elusive.

Earlier CDS data indicated that the quality and completeness of recovery from an MDD episode are associated with a highly significant delay in episode relapse (Judd et al. 1998b) and reduced overall future course chronicity (Judd et al. 2000b). In 237 patients who met RDC for remission from their index MDEs, survival analysis showed a significantly slower time to relapse for those who recovered completely symptom free (asymptomatic recovery), compared with those who recovered with ongoing residual subsyndromal depressive symptoms (residual symptom recovery) (Judd et al. 1998b). The group who recovered to the asymptomatic status remained free of *any* type of depressive episode (major, minor, or dysthymic) 5.6 times longer than did the group who recovered with residual symptoms (median = 184 vs. 33 weeks, respectively; $P < 0.001$) (Figure 3–3). Patients with asymptomatic recovery remained free of a subsequent MDE 3.4 times longer than did those who recovered and retained residual symptoms (median time to next MDE onset = 231 vs. 68 weeks, respectively; $P < 0.001$). There was no evidence that the more rapid relapse in the residual symptom recovery group was attributable to less intense treatment with antidepressants; in fact, these patients received significantly more antidepressant treatment during the recovery interval than did the asymptomatic group.

A previous investigation of the CDS cohort (Keller et al. 1983b) found that a history of more than three MDEs was the strongest predictor of early MDE relapse described up to that point in time. However, a subsequent investigation (Judd et al. 1998b) showed that the presence of ongoing residual subthreshold depressive symptoms following resolution of an MDE was a stronger predictor of early depressive episode relapse than was the more than three prior episodes risk factor. The odds ratio for risk of relapse for each risk factor, after controlling for the other, was 3.64 for recovery status compared with 1.64 for more than three prior episodes. In fact, a history of more than three compared with zero to three prior MDEs was significantly associated with early relapse *only* within the asymptomatic recovery group (median = 79 vs. 274 weeks, respectively; $P < 0.001$). The recurrent MDE risk factor had little effect on time to relapse among the residual symptom recovery patients; in fact, the survival curves for more than three compared with zero to three prior episodes were nearly superimposed on each other (median = 28 vs. 34 weeks, respectively; $P = 0.283$).

A subsequent survival analysis was conducted on the time to next MDE relapse in 96 of the CDS patients who were recovering from their *first lifetime MDE* (Judd et al. 2000b). Among these first-MDE patients, those with asymptomatic recovery remained episode free almost four times longer before experiencing a relapse than did those who recovered with residual depressive symptoms (median = 384 vs. 103 weeks, respectively; $P < 0.001$). Not only was residual symptom recovery associated with significantly faster MDE relapse, but the future course of illness for these subjects was significantly more severe and chronic, as follows: they experienced a 2.4 times higher odds for depressive episode relapse during any given week of follow-up; significantly fewer asymptomatic weeks during the next 10 years (31.8% weeks vs. 78.7% weeks, respectively; $P < 0.001$); significantly more MDEs during their future course of illness ($P = 0.006$); and significantly shorter interepisode well intervals during the remainder of follow-up (median = 22 vs. 154 weeks, respectively; $P = 0.001$).

Although the optimal definition of MDD recovery remains uncertain (Dunlop et al. 2012), these findings from the CDS indicate that resolution of

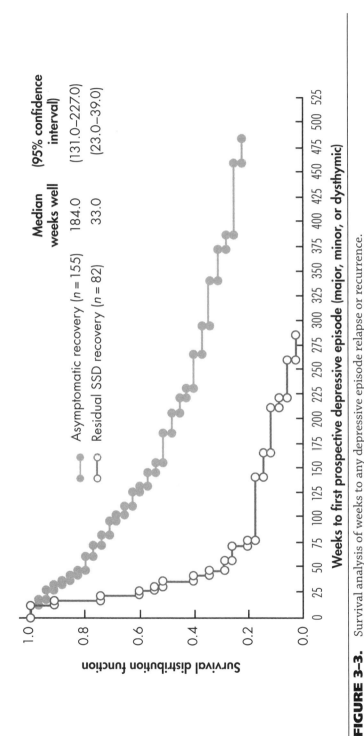

	Median weeks well	(95% confidence interval)
— Asymptomatic recovery (n = 155)	184.0	(131.0–227.0)
○ Residual SSD recovery (n = 82)	33.0	(23.0–39.0)

FIGURE 3–3. Survival analysis of weeks to any depressive episode relapse or recurrence.

Collaborative Depression Study patients with unipolar major depressive disorder who recovered from the intake major depressive episode with residual subsyndromal depressive symptoms were compared with patients who had asymptomatic status. Wilcoxon χ^2 test of overall difference = 80.29; $P < 0.001$. SSD = subsyndromal depressive symptoms (below minor depression/dysthymia threshold).

Source. Reprinted from Judd LL, Akiskal HS, Maser JD, et al.: "Major Depressive Disorder: A Prospective Study of Residual Subthreshold Depressive Symptoms as a Predictor of Rapid Relapse." *Journal of Affective Disorders* 50:97–108, 1998. Copyright Elsevier 1998. Used with permission.

MDEs with ongoing residual subthreshold depressive symptoms, even following the first lifetime episode, appears to be the first step in a significantly more severe, relapsing, and chronic future course of illness. When ongoing residual subsyndromal symptoms continue after resolution of an acute MDE, full MDE remission or recovery has *not* been achieved, the MDE is still active, resolution is incomplete, psychosocial function is significantly impaired, and the subject is at heightened risk for a rapid episode relapse. Consistent with this idea is that sleep neurophysiological indices of depression such as shortened rapid eye movement (REM) sleep latency and increased REM density are present at minor, dysthymic, and residual phases of MDD, indicating that the illness is biologically active at all symptom levels of depression (Akiskal et al. 1997).

These data indicate that treatment is needed as long as *any* depressive symptoms are present, and ongoing treatment should be considered until asymptomatic recovery is achieved. Full resolution of residual subsyndromal depressive symptoms may require higher doses, different classes, or combinations of antidepressant medication; augmentation with mood stabilizers; or depression-specific psychotherapy. Prospective, controlled treatment studies are needed to determine whether all patients with MDE can be treated to the asymptomatic status and which therapeutic strategies are most effective in achieving this goal. Examination of clinical and biological moderators may indicate subsets of patients for whom particular treatment approaches are optimal.

These findings raise questions about the long-standing practice of researchers and clinicians to consider that an MDE is essentially remitted or recovered when minimal subsyndromal depressive symptoms are still present. It now appears that true MDE recovery is achieved only when all signs and symptoms of depressive episodes abate and the subject is asymptomatic for a sufficient time to reach a stable state of recovery.

Summary of Findings Based on the Dimensional Paradigm of Major Depressive Disorder

The prospective follow-up of patients in the CDS provides a comprehensive picture of the long-term course of unipolar MDD. MDD is a common and primarily chronic illness, with powerful tendencies for major, minor, or dysthymic depressive episodes to relapse or recur during the subject's lifetime. Patients are symptomatic from the illness with varying levels of depressive symptom severity most of the time (mean = 55.4% of weeks) during long-term follow-up. For purposes of diagnosis, MDD is a categorical illness, with well-defined boundaries for the onset of episodes; however, the longitudinal symptomatic expression of MDD is characterized by a dimensional continuum of depressive symptom severity that includes major, minor or dysthymic, and subsyndromal depression. The typical course is dynamic and fluctuating, with various levels of depressive symptom severity alternating within the same subject. The symptomatic periods are sporadically interspersed with periods when the subject is asymptomatic (euthymic); only then is the illness inactive.

Although much of the clinical and research focus has been to characterize and manage acute MDEs, subjects with MDD are longitudinally symptomatic at the minor and subsyndromal depressive symptom severity levels 2.7 times more often than at the diagnostic threshold for major depression. Every increment in depressive symptom severity is associated with a significant stepwise increase in psychosocial disability. This is consistent with the proposition that the threshold for detecting clinically relevant depressive illness in someone who has experienced an MDE should include *all levels* of depressive symptom severity. The presence of ongoing residual subsyndromal depressive symptoms following MDE resolution, even though it may meet current definitions of MDE recovery, indicates that an MDE is still clinically active and unremitted, the patient is at risk for early episode relapse, significant psychosocial impairment is likely to be present, and continued treatment is warranted. These data strongly suggest that full MDE resolution should be defined by the abatement of *all* depressive symptoms for a sufficient time for the patient to enter a stable state of recovery.

Clinical Implications

- Major depressive disorder (MDD) should be treated as primarily a chronic, often lifelong illness, with powerful tendencies for depressive episodes to relapse and recur. The first goal of treatment is amelioration of the symptoms of an acute depressive episode, but long-term follow-up by a clinician or case manager should be provided on a periodic or as-needed basis.
- Patients, their families, and others who are part of their support system need to be given scientifically accurate information about the strong tendencies for episode relapse and recurrence; early warning signs or symptoms of an impending episode and the need to contact the clinician at the first of these signs; the need for strict adherence to the recommended therapeutic regimen;

and the importance of bringing any treatment compliance problems to the attention of the clinician.

- Every level of severity of depressive symptoms in MDD, including subsyndromal symptoms, needs to be a treatment target because the presence of *any* depressive symptom indicates that the illness is active, psychosocial dysfunction is present, and the risk for relapse or recurrence is high.

- The clinician's immediate goal is aggressive management of the acute episode with evidence-based treatments (antidepressant and other medications as well as psychotherapy) to achieve the abatement of *all* depressive symptoms and maintain the asymptomatic status until a stable state of full episode recovery is achieved.

- As with all chronic illnesses, the ultimate long-term goal with the MDD patient is to reduce chronicity, prevent exacerbations and recurrences, and maintain the patient as symptom free as possible, with optimal psychosocial functioning, throughout his or her lifetime.

References

Akiskal HS: Dysthymic disorder: psychopathology of proposed chronic depressive subtypes. Am J Psychiatry 140:11–20, 1983

Akiskal HS: Dysthymic and cyclothymic depressions: therapeutic considerations. J Clin Psychiatry 55(suppl):46–52, 1994

Akiskal HS, Judd LL, Gillin JC, et al: Subthreshold depressions: clinical and polysomnographic validation of dysthymic, residual and masked forms. J Affect Disord 45:53–63, 1997

American Psychiatric Association: Diagnostic and Statistical Manual of Mental Disorders, 3rd Edition. Washington, DC, American Psychiatric Association, 1980

American Psychiatric Association: Diagnostic and Statistical Manual of Mental Disorders, 4th Edition, Text Revision. Washington, DC, American Psychiatric Association, 2000

Angst J, Preisig M: Course of a clinical cohort of unipolar, bipolar and schizoaffective patients: results of a prospective study from 1959 to 1985. Schweiz Arch Neurol Psychiatr 146:5–16, 1995

Angst J, Gamma A, Sellaro R, et al: Recurrence of bipolar disorders and major depression: a life-long perspective. Eur Arch Psychiatry Clin Neurosci 253:236–240, 2003

Brodaty H, Luscombe G, Peisah C, et al: A 25-year longitudinal, comparison study of the outcome of depression. Psychol Med 31:1347–1359, 2001

Coryell W, Endicott J, Keller M: Outcome of patients with chronic affective disorders: a five year follow-up. Am J Psychiatry 47:1627–1633, 1990

Coryell W, Solomon D, Leon A, et al: Does major depressive disorder change with age? Psychol Med 39:1689–1695, 2009

Dunlop BW, Holland P, Bao W, et al: Recovery and subsequent recurrence in patients with recurrent major depressive disorder. J Psychiatr Res 46:708–715, 2012

Greenfield S, Ware J: The functioning and well-being of depressed patients: results from the Medical Outcomes Study. JAMA 262:914–919, 1989

Hoencamp E, Haffmans PM, Griens AM, et al: A 3.5-year naturalistic follow-up study of depressed out-patients. J Affect Disord 66:267–271, 2001

Judd LL: Pleomorphic expressions of unipolar depressive disease: summary of the 1996 CINP President's Workshop. J Affect Disord 45:109–116, 1997

Judd LL, Rapaport MH, Paulus MP, et al: Subsyndromal symptomatic depression (SSD): a new mood disorder? J Clin Psychiatry 55:18S–28S, 1994

Judd LL, Paulus MB, Wells KB, et al: Socioeconomic burden of subsyndromal depressive symptoms and major depression in a sample of the general population. Am J Psychiatry 153:1411–1417, 1996

Judd LL, Akiskal HS, Paulus MP: The role and clinical significance of subsyndromal depressive symptoms (SSD) in unipolar major depressive disorder. J Affect Disord 45:5–18, 1997a

Judd LL, Paulus M, Akiskal HS, et al: The role of subsyndromal depressive symptoms in unipolar major depression, in Basic and Clinical Science of Mental and Addictive Disorder. Edited by Judd LL, Saletu B, Filip V. Basel, Switzerland, Karger Press, 1997b, pp 6–10

Judd LL, Akiskal HS, Maser JD, et al: A prospective 12-year study of subsyndromal and syndromal depressive symptoms in unipolar major depressive disorders. Arch Gen Psychiatry 55:694–700, 1998a

Judd LL, Akiskal HS, Maser JD, et al: Major depressive disorder: a prospective study of residual subthreshold depressive symptoms as a predictor of rapid relapse. J Affect Disord 50:97–108, 1998b

Judd LL, Akiskal HS, Zeller PJ, et al: Psychosocial disability during the long-term course of unipolar major depressive disorder. Arch Gen Psychiatry 57:375–380, 2000a

Judd LL, Paulus MP, Zeller PJ, et al: Does incomplete recovery from first lifetime major depressive episode herald a chronic course of illness? Am J Psychiatry 157:1501–1504, 2000b

Judd LL, Schettler PJ, Akiskal HS: The prevalence, clinical relevance and public health significance of subthreshold depressive symptoms. Psychiatr Clin North Am 25:685–698, 2002

Katz MM, Klerman GL: Introduction: overview of the clinical studies program. Am J Psychiatry 136:49–51, 1979

Katz MM, Secunda SK, Hirschfeld RMA, et al: NIMH Clinical Research Branch Collaborative Program on the Psychobiology of Depression. Arch Gen Psychiatry 36:765–771, 1979

Keller MB, Lavori PW, Endicott J, et al: "Double depression": two-year follow-up. Am J Psychiatry 140:689–694, 1983a

Keller MB, Lavori PW, Lewis CE, et al: Predictors of relapse in major depressive disorder. JAMA 250:3299–3304, 1983b

Keller M, Lavori P, Friedman B, et al: Longitudinal interval follow-up evaluation. Arch Gen Psychiatry 44:540–548, 1987

Keller MB, Lavori PW, Mueller TI, et al: Time to recovery, chronicity, and levels of psy-chopathology in major depression: a 5-year prospective follow-up of 431 sub-jects. Arch Gen Psychiatry 49:809–816, 1992

Kessler RC, Birnbaum H, Bromet E, et al: Age differences in major depression: results from the National Comorbidity Survey Replication (NCS-R). Psychol Med 40:225–237, 2010

Kovacs M, Akiskal HS, Gatsonis C, et al: Childhood-onset dysthymic disorder: clinical features and prospective naturalistic outcome. Arch Gen Psychiatry 51:365–374, 1994

Mueller TI, Leon AC, Keller MB, et al: Recurrence after recovery from major depressive disorder during 15 years of observational follow-up. Am J Psychiatry 156:1000–1006, 1999

Spitzer RL, Endicott J, Robins E: Research Diagnostic Criteria for a Selected Group of Functional Disorders, 3rd Edition. New York, New York Biometrics Research Di-vision, New York State Psychiatric Institute, 1977

Wakefield JC: Disorder as harmful dysfunction: a conceptual critique of DSM-III-R's definition of mental disorder. Psychol Rev 99:232–247, 1992

Weissman MM, Leaf PJ, Tischler GL, et al: Affective disorders in five United States communities. Psychol Med 18:141–153, 1988

World Health Organization: The ICD-10 Classification of Mental and Behavioural Dis-orders: Clinical Descriptions and Diagnostic Guidelines. Geneva, Switzerland, World Health Organization, 1992

CHAPTER 4

Dimensional Symptomatic Structure of the Long-Term Course of Bipolar I and Bipolar II Disorders

Lewis L. Judd, M.D.

Pamela J. Schettler, Ph.D.

Hagop S. Akiskal, M.D.

Martin B. Keller, M.D.

IN THIS CHAPTER we present the results of a series of studies that used a dimensional paradigm of symptom severity and polarity to describe the long-term course of illness for patients with bipolar disorders in the National Institute of Mental Health (NIMH) Collaborative Depression Study (CDS). Results of our dimensional analyses of the long-term course of unipolar major depressive disorder (MDD) (Judd et al. 1998a, 1998b, 2000a, 2000b) are presented in Chapter 3 ("Dimensional Symptomatic Structure of the Long-Term Course of Unipolar Major Depressive Disorder") of this volume. Following our work on unipolar MDD, we carried out a parallel series of studies of patients with bipolar disorders (Judd et al. 2002, 2003a, 2003b, 2003c, 2005, 2008a, 2008b), the results of which have been summarized previously (Judd and Schettler 2010). The purpose of these studies was to fill the enormous gap in empirical data concerning the long-term course and the life effects of bipolar I and bipolar II disorders. The findings presented here have strong implications for how bipolar illnesses should be managed over time. Recommendations for long-term clinical management of bipolar disorders are presented at the conclusion of this chapter.

Methods

Findings presented here are based on the bipolar disorder cohort of the NIMH CDS (Katz and Klerman 1979; Katz et al. 1979). The CDS was unique in that it obtained prospective, naturalistic, systematic, long-term follow-up data on the weekly symptom status of a very large cohort of patients with mood disorders diagnosed with research-based criteria. Patients entered the study in a major affective episode, from 1978 to 1981. Findings reported in this chapter were derived from data extending up to 30 years of follow-up, with an average of 19 years per subject, for 214 patients with bipolar I or II disorder.

Subjects

Methods for diagnosis and follow-up of CDS subjects have been described in Chapter 2 ("Collaborative Depression Study Procedures and Study Design") of this volume. Patients were included in the current analysis if their symptoms met criteria for bipolar I (definite) or bipolar II (definite or probable) disorder at entry. Because we found no difference in clinical, demographic, or follow-up characteristics between patients with bipolar II disorder who had hypomanic episodes lasting 1 week or more (definite bipolar II disorder) and those with episodes lasting 3–6 days (probable bipolar II disorder) (Judd et al. 2003b), we combined both groups into the bipolar II cohort. To focus on possible confounding diagnoses, we excluded 38 patients whose symptoms had ever met Research Diagnostic Criteria (Spitzer et al. 1977) for schizophrenia or schizoaffective disorder, as well as 28 with an unstable diagnosis (bipolar II to bipolar I disorder) during follow-up and 25 patients whose symptoms did not meet DSM-IV-TR bipolar disorder criteria (American Psychiatric Association 2000) because they had no MDD by the end of follow-up. Interview forms rated with poor or very poor reliability of weekly symptom status were omitted from the analysis (3% of follow-up forms, accounting for 6% of follow-up weeks). Finally, to focus on the long-term course of bipolar disorders, 36 subjects with less than 2 years of reliable data for weekly symptom status (10.8% of those qualifying on the basis of diagnosis) were excluded. The resulting analysis sample included 139 patients with bipolar I disorder (lifetime MDD and mania) and 75 patients with bipolar II disorder (lifetime MDD and hypomania but no mania). Demographic and clinical characteristics and length of follow-up are shown in Table 4–1. Half of the subjects (50.9%) were followed up for 20–30 years.

TABLE 4–1. Demographic and clinical characteristics and length of prospective follow-up for Collaborative Depression Study (CDS) patients with bipolar I or II disorder and 2–30 years of follow-up data

	Bipolar I (*n*=139)	Bipolar II (*n*=75)	Significance
Intake characteristics			
Demographics			
Age (years, mean [SD; range])	40.4 [15.5; 17–79]	39.9 [15.7; 18–76]	$t_{212}=0.224$; $P=0.823$
Female gender (*n* [%])	84 [60.4]	47 [62.7]	$\chi^2_1=0.102$; $P=0.749$
Education—some college (*n* [%])	71 [51.1]	38 [50.7]	$\chi^2_1=0.003$; $P=0.954$
Marital status[a] (*n* [%])			$\chi^2_2=0.773$
Married/living together	57 [41.0]	35 [46.7]	$P=0.680$
Separated/widowed/ divorced	36 [25.9]	19 [25.3]	
Never married	46 [33.1]	21 [28.0]	
Episode history			
Age at onset of first affective episode (years, mean [SD; range])	27.5 [14.1; 6–72]	27.8 [13.9; 12–68]	$t_{212}=0.149$; $P=0.882$
Onset of first affective episode before age 21 (*n* [%])	53 [38.1]	28 [37.3]	$\chi^2_1=0.013$; $P=0.909$
Number of lifetime affective episodes (including intake) (*n* [%])			$\chi^2_2=0.802$; $P=0.670$
1 (first episode)	27 [19.4]	18 [24.0]	
2 or 3	53 [38.1]	29 [38.7]	
≥4	59 [42.4]	28 [37.3]	

TABLE 4–1. Demographic and clinical characteristics and length of prospective follow-up for Collaborative Depression Study (CDS) patients with bipolar I or II disorder and 2–30 years of follow-up data *(continued)*

	Bipolar I (n=139)	Bipolar II (n=75)	Significance
Clinical characteristics			
Inpatient status (n [%])	116 [83.5]	62 [82.7]	$\chi^2_1=0.022$; $P=0.883$
Global Assessment Scale (GAS) for worst period in episode[b] (mean [SD])	36.5 [10.8]	39.9 [11.0]	$t_{212}=2.183$; $P=0.030$
Psychotic features in intake episode (n [%])	24 [17.3]	9 [12.0]	$\chi^2_1=1.036$; $P=0.309$
Length of CDS follow-up (years)			$t_{212}=0.228$; $P=0.820$
Mean (SD)	18. (9.1)	19.0 (9.4)	
Median	19.8	20.4	
Range	2–30	2–30	
2–9 (n [%])	28 [20.1]	17 [22.7]	
10–19 (n [%])	42 [30.3]	18 [24.0]	
20–30 (n [%])	69 [49.6]	40 [53.3]	

Note. Patients who entered the CDS with a diagnosis of bipolar I disorder (definite) or bipolar II disorder (probable or definite) with no evidence of schizoaffective disorder or schizophrenia by the end of CDS follow-up. Analysis of long-term follow-up course is based on subjects with at least 2 years (104 weeks) of follow-up data rated "fair" or better in terms of accuracy (i.e., excluding weeks deemed to have "poor" or "very poor" data).
[a]Marital status information is missing for two subjects.
[b]GAS score measures severity of symptoms and impairment. Scores range from 1 (most severe and impaired) to 100 (superior functioning with no symptoms). A mean of approaching 40 represents major impairment in several areas, or some impairment in reality testing or communication, or at least one suicide attempt.

Affective Symptom Polarity and Severity Categories

For the analyses reported here, each week's psychiatric symptom ratings on all affective conditions, from all variations of Longitudinal Interval Follow-Up Evaluation interviews (Keller et al. 1987) used from intake to final follow-up as described in Chapter 2, were combined and classified into one of eight mutually exclusive weekly symptom status categories (see Table 4–2). These include three levels of severity of symptoms in the pure depressive spectrum—major depression (MDD), minor depression or dysthymia, and subsyndromal depression—and three levels of symptom severity in the pure manic spectrum—mania, hypomania, and subsyndromal hypomania. A separate category includes both cycling (changing polarity) and mixed polarity (concurrent manic and depressive spectrum symptoms) within a given week. The final category is the asymptomatic status (no affective symptoms; return to usual self).

Findings

Symptomatic Chronicity of the Course of Bipolar Illness

The field considers bipolar disorders to be primarily chronic illnesses because of their very high likelihood of relapse and recurrence of affective episodes. However, a unique picture of just how chronic these disorders really are emerges from our studies based on the weekly psychiatric status ratings. A new measure of chronicity, which we have been advocating for the study of both unipolar MDD and bipolar disorders, is the total percentage of weeks when subjects experience *any* level of affective symptoms from their illness (i.e., the percentage of course that the illness is active). The total time symptomatic is a broader indicator of illness chronicity than is time in affective episodes because patients with bipolar (and unipolar) disorder, even when consensus criteria for "recovery" are met, frequently retain subsyndromal affective symptoms (Judd et al. 1998b, 2008b). As shown in Table 4–3, patients with bipolar I disorder were symptomatic from their illness during a mean of 53.2% of follow-up weeks, and patients with bipolar II disorder were symptomatic 49.4% of the time. Thus, both bipolar I and II disorders are highly chronic, with patients being afflicted by an active state of the illness approximately half of the time during up to 30 years of systematic follow-up. As expected, the proposed alternative measure of chronicity is substantially higher than the mean percentage of time the same subjects spent in affective episodes during 2–30 years of follow-up, which was 40.7% and 34.2% for those with bipolar I and II disorders, respectively.

TABLE 4–2. Classification of affective symptom severity levels based on weekly psychiatric status rating (PSR) scale scores across all four groups of affective disorders

Affective symptom severity level	Major depressive disorder (MDD) or mania (6-point PSR scale)[a]	Minor depression/ hypomania (3-point PSR scale)[b]	DSM-III depressive conditions[c] (3-point PSR scale)[b]	RDC cyclothymic personality (3-point PSR scale)[b]
1 Asymptomatic: no depressive or manic spectrum symptoms of the episode; return to usual self	1	1	1	1
2 Subsyndromal: depressive spectrum symptoms *below* MinD level or subsyndromal manic spectrum symptoms below hypomania level	1	1	2 or 3	2 or 3
	1	2	(Any)[d]	(Any)
	2	1 or 2	(Any)	(Any)
3 Affective symptoms at the MinD/dysthymia or hypomania level	1	3	(Any)	(Any)
	2	3	(Any)	(Any)
	3	(Any)	(Any)	(Any)
	4	(Any)	(Any)	(Any)
4 Affective symptoms at the MDD or mania level	5	(Any)	(Any)	(Any)
	6	(Any)	(Any)	(Any)

Note. Weekly symptom severity level is assigned based on each week's ratings on all affective conditions regardless of whether the patient was in a Research Diagnostic Criteria (RDC) episode at that time. Rated affective conditions include RDC MDD; RDC minor or intermittent depressive or dysthymic disorder (MinD); RDC hypomanic disorder; RDC cyclothymic personality; and DSM-III (American Psychiatric Association 1980) atypical depression (code 296.82) and adjustment disorder with depressed mood (code 309.00). Weekly symptom severity levels are mutually exclusive. Read across the table for combinations of PSR values that result in classifying a particular week at a given symptom severity level. For example, a patient would be classified at the minor depression or dysthymia level for the week he or she was rated as PSR 3 or 4 on the 6-point major depression scale, or PSR 3 on the 3-point minor depression or dysthymia scale with a PSR 1 or 2 on the 6-point major depression scale.

[a]6-Point weekly PSR scale values: 1 = asymptomatic, returned to usual self; 2 = residual/mild affective symptoms; 3 = partial remission, moderate symptoms or impairment; 4 = marked or major symptoms or impairment; 5 = definite criteria without prominent psychotic symptoms or extreme impairment; 6 = definite criteria with prominent psychotic symptoms or extreme impairment.

[b]3-Point weekly PSR scale values: 1 = asymptomatic, returned to usual self; 2 = probable criteria (mild symptoms); 3 = definite criteria (severe symptoms).

[c]Includes DSM-III atypical depression (code 296.82) and adjustment disorder with depressed mood (code 309.00).

[d]"(Any)" indicates any PSR value of this affective condition qualifies for the given symptom severity level, in conjunction with the values shown for other affective conditions. For example, a given week is classified at the MDD level based on a PSR value of 5 or 6 for MDD regardless of PSR values on any other affective condition(s).

TABLE 4–3. Percentage of weeks spent in affective symptom polarity and severity categories during long-term prospective follow-up for Collaborative Depression Study patients with bipolar I or II disorder and 2–30 years of follow-up data

Affective symptom polarity/severity category	Bipolar I [mean (SD); $n=139$]	Bipolar II [mean (SD); $n=75$]	Significance[a] (t; P)
Asymptomatic (no affective symptoms)	46.8 (33.7)	50.6 (34.1)	0.87_{212}; 0.385
Symptomatic (any affective symptoms)	53.2 (33.7)	49.4 (34.1)	0.87_{212}; 0.385
Symptoms by mutually exclusive polarity/severity categories			
Pure depression (no manic symptoms)	46.9 (34.2)	49.2 (34.1)	0.16_{212}; 0.876
Subsyndromal depressive symptoms	14.1 (17.0)	16.3 (18.5)	1.14_{212}; 0.258
Minor depression/dysthymia threshold	20.0 (20.7)	21.2 (22.0)	0.32_{212}; 0.750
Major depressive disorder threshold	12.8 (19.2)	11.8 (16.0)	0.17_{212}; 0.864
Pure mania/hypomania (no depression symptoms)	2.9 (8.4)	0.1 (0.4)	$3.92_{139.2}{}^{b}$; <0.001
Subsyndromal hypomanic symptoms	0.6 (2.9)	0.01 (0.02)	$3.99_{142.6}{}^{b}$; <0.001
Hypomania threshold	1.6 (5.8)	0.1 (0.4)	$4.06_{165}{}^{b}$; <0.001
Mania threshold	0.7 (2.4)	—	—
Cycling/mixed polarity (all severity levels)	3.4 (9.8)	0.1 (0.5)	$3.51_{139}{}^{b}$; <0.001

TABLE 4–3. Percentage of weeks spent in affective symptom polarity and severity categories during long-term prospective follow-up for Collaborative Depression Study patients with bipolar I or II disorder and 2–30 years of follow-up data *(continued)*

Affective symptom polarity/severity category	Bipolar I [mean (SD); $n=139$]	Bipolar II [mean (SD); $n=75$]	Significance[a] (t; P)
Symptoms by polarity			
Any level of depressive symptoms	50.3 (34.3)	49.3 (34.1)	0.51_{212}; 0.613
Any level of manic spectrum symptoms	6.3 (14.7)	0.2 (0.6)	$6.52_{66.4}$[b]; <0.001
Symptoms by severity level/threshold			
Subthreshold depression/hypomania	15.7 (17.1)	16.3 (18.4)	0.25_{212}; 0.799
Minor depression/dysthymia/hypomanic	23.1 (21.7)	21.3 (22.0)	0.86_{212}; 0.393
Major depression/mania	13.3 (19.1)	11.8 (16.1)	1.10_{212}; 0.272

[a]Percentages were compared after arcsine transformation.
[b]Satterthwaite adjustment to degrees of freedom, for unequal group variances.

Dimensional Expression of Affective Symptom Severity Levels

Over the long-term course, affective symptoms in bipolar disorder are expressed along a dimensional continuum of progressively increasing symptom severity, ranging from subsyndromal through symptoms at the threshold for minor depression, dysthymia, or hypomania to symptoms at the full syndromal threshold of mania and major depressive episodes (MDEs). Table 4–3 and Figure 4–1 show the mean percentage of weeks of follow-up that subjects with bipolar I and II disorders spent in each of eight mutually exclusive symptom severity categories: three levels of depressive symptom severity, three levels of manic or hypomanic symptom severity, symptoms of mixed polarity, or the asymptomatic status. A great majority of these bipolar patients experienced the full range of symptom severity of both depressive and manic symptoms during their highly dynamic long-term course of illness. The design of the CDS, with its record of weekly affective symptom status, provides a unique picture of the long-term symptomatic course of bipolar disorders.

Dominance of Affective Symptoms Below Syndromal Threshold of Major Depression and Mania

As can be seen in Table 4–3, most of the symptomatic course of both bipolar I and II disorders occurs below the syndromal threshold for MDE and mania. Even though bipolar disorder is traditionally defined by episodes at the syndromal threshold of major depression or mania, CDS patients spent only about one-third as much time at those syndromal symptom levels during their long-term course (mean = 14.4% for bipolar I and 11.8% for bipolar II disorder) as at mild or moderate levels of affective symptom severity (mean = 38.8% for bipolar I and 37.6% for bipolar II disorder).

Subsyndromal manic symptoms are particularly important during bipolar MDEs. As we have found (Judd et al. 2012), 76% of intake MDEs in CDS patients with bipolar disorder included concurrent subsyndromal hypomanic symptoms, and this was a marker of a more severe form of bipolar illness marked by greater suicidality, disability, and comorbidity. This finding is consistent with other findings from the NIMH Systematic Treatment Enhancement Program for Bipolar Disorder study (Goldberg et al. 2009) and other research groups (Akiskal and Benazzi 2005; Balázs et al. 2006; Hawton et al. 2005). Subsyndromal manic symptoms are also an important factor in medication decisions. Antidepressants are used frequently to treat bipolar depression—typically as an adjunct to mood stabilizers to minimize the risk of manic

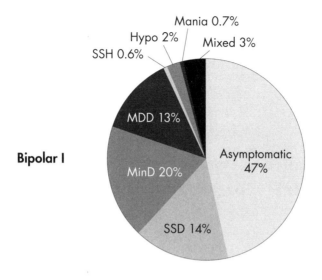

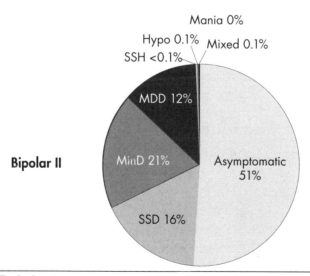

FIGURE 4–1. Mean percentage of weeks in each category of affective symptom severity during long-term follow-up (median = 20 years) of Collaborative Depression Study patients with bipolar disorder.

Asymptomatic = no symptoms of the affective episode (usual self); Hypo = hypomania threshold; Mania = manic episode threshold; MDD = major depressive episode threshold; MinD = minor depression/dysthymia threshold; Mixed = concurrent symptoms of depressive and manic/hypomanic polarity; SSD = subsyndromal depressive symptoms (below MinD threshold); SSH = subsyndromal hypomanic symptoms (below hypomania threshold).

or hypomanic switches resulting from antidepressant use alone. The efficacy of specific antidepressants, and the characteristics of individuals who are most likely to benefit from such adjunctive treatment, is an important area of current research (Salvi et al. 2008). Some evidence indicates that when concurrent subsyndromal manic symptoms are present (arguably a form of mixed state), the use of adjunctive treatment with antidepressants increases the risk of exacerbating the manic symptoms, while not hastening recovery from the acute bipolar MDE (Frye et al. 2009; Goldberg et al. 2007).

Dominance of Depression Over Mania or Hypomania

A very high prevalence of depressive episodes and symptoms occurs over the long-term course of bipolar illness. When all levels of symptom severity in each spectrum were combined (Table 4–3), patients with bipolar I disorder experienced eight times more depression than mania or hypomania during long-term follow-up (50.3% vs. 6.3% of weeks). The long-term symptomatic course of bipolar II disorder was almost exclusively depressive (49.3% of weeks), with hypomanic or subsyndromal hypomanic symptoms reported during only 0.2% of follow-up weeks. As discussed later in this chapter, manic spectrum symptoms may be underreported by patients with bipolar II disorder. Nevertheless, these findings provide striking evidence that effective management of depressive episodes and symptoms remains a pressing challenge for bipolar disorders.

Dynamic and Changeable Symptomatic Course of Bipolar Illness

Angst and colleagues reported that patients with bipolar II disorder experience a slightly higher number of episodes per year than do patients with bipolar I disorder (Angst and Preisig 1995; Angst et al. 2003b). In an article based on the CDS, Judd et al. (2003a) confirmed and extended these findings by comparing patients with bipolar I disorder with those with bipolar II disorder on the number, duration, and percentage of weeks spent in each type of affective episode during a 10-year period after the end of their intake episode. Both bipolar groups spent about 30% of that time in major or minor mood disorder episodes. Patients with bipolar II disorder tended to have more episodes (mean [SD] = 4.2 [2.6] vs. 3.3 [2.5]; $P = 0.052$), including significantly more episodes of major depression and of minor depression or dysthymia. Patients with bipolar I disorder, on the contrary, had significantly more episodes with cycling or mixed polarity. During this 10-year period, the duration of each type of episode was slightly (nonsignificantly) longer for patients with bipolar II than for those with bipolar I disorder. The episodic course of bipolar disorders in CDS patients is covered in much more detail in Chapter 13 ("Predictors of Course and Outcome of Bipolar Disorder") of this volume.

When data on episode status are supplemented with analysis of week-to-week change in affective symptom severity or polarity, the results show a strikingly high number of changes in symptom status per year in bipolar disorder. The mean total number of changes per year in symptom status (symptom severity and polarity) overall of long-term follow-up (2–31 years) was 3.6 in bipolar I disorder and 1.8 in bipolar II disorder (see Table 4–4). In Chapter 3 of this volume, we report that unipolar MDD patients in the CDS changed depressive symptom severity level a mean of 1.5 times per year. This corroborates Angst's findings of greater change in bipolar disorder compared with unipolar disorder (Angst and Preisig 1995; Angst et al. 2003b). Shifts per year in symptom *polarity* are defined by a patient shifting from symptoms in the depressive spectrum to those in the manic spectrum or vice versa, with or without an intervening asymptomatic period. On average, bipolar I patients moved between mania or hypomania and depression 1.9 times per year, whereas bipolar II patients reported an average of only 0.1 polarity changes per year. Findings based on shifts in polarity and severity of affective symptoms add to our understanding based on episode status and support the idea that, although equal in symptomatic chronicity, bipolar I disorder may be the more dynamic and changeable of the two disorders, whereas bipolar II disorder is characterized by more frequent episodes.

Psychosocial Impairment Associated With Bipolar Disorders

When we examined global psychosocial disability averaged across all ill and well periods during their long-term course (Judd et al. 2008b), mean levels of global functioning for patients with bipolar I or II disorder reflected a mild level of impairment. Both groups experienced *some* degree of impairment during nearly 60% of the months during follow-up (58.3% for bipolar I; 59.1% for bipolar II), which included *moderate to severe* impairment during 30% of follow-up months (31.3% for bipolar I; 30.3% for bipolar II). Impairment for both bipolar groups was slightly higher than for patients with unipolar MDD, who experienced 53.8% of months with some impairment, and 25.8% had moderate to severe impairment during long-term follow-up.

Data summarized in this section are from the first investigation of which we are aware to study psychosocial impairment associated with *every* level of affective symptom severity and periods of euthymia in a large cohort of bipolar I and II patients followed up prospectively for many years (Judd et al. 2005). In Figure 4–2, mean ratings of global psychosocial impairment associated with months spent in each symptom status category are shown. As seen

TABLE 4–4. Symptom status and polarity changes during long-term prospective follow-up for Collaborative Depression Study patients with bipolar I or II disorder and 2–30 years of follow-up data

	Bipolar I (n=139)	Bipolar II (n=75)	Significance (Wilcoxon rank sum; P)
Changes in symptom severity or polarity			
Changes per year (mean [SD; range])	3.6 [5.3; 0.1–34.5]	1.8 [1.7; [0.1–9.2]	0.040
Mean ≥ 5 changes per year (n [%])	26 (18.7)	4 (5.3)	$\chi^2_1 = 6.160$; $P = 0.013$
Changes in polarity			
Changes per year (mean [SD; range])	1.9 [5.1; 0.0–32.8]	0.10 [0.3; 0.0–1.9]	0.002
Mean ≥ 2 changes per year (n [%])	24 [17.3]	0 [0.0]	$\chi^2_1 = 12.903$; $P < 0.001$

in the figure, affective symptom severity and psychosocial impairment fluctuate together within the individual patient during the course of bipolar illness. The figure clearly shows that depressive symptoms, which dominate the course of both bipolar disorders, are at least as impairing as symptoms of comparable severity in the manic or hypomanic spectrum. Every stepwise increase or decrease in depressive symptom severity is linked to a parallel, statistically significant, stepwise increase or decrease in psychosocial impairment in both bipolar I and II disorder. When subjects with either disorder are asymptomatic, psychosocial functioning is rated as good. When the same patients are experiencing subsyndromal depressive symptoms, they have mild impairment. During months with symptoms at the level of minor depression or dysthymia, their psychosocial impairment is rated as significantly worse, between mild and moderate, and when bipolar patients are experiencing symptoms at the syndromal threshold of major depression, their psychosocial functioning is rated as moderately impaired. Note that even subsyndromal depressive symptoms are associated with significantly more impairment than is the asymptomatic (euthymic) status for both bipolar I and bipolar II disorder.

For patients with bipolar I disorder, a similar picture of a stepwise increase or decrease in psychosocial impairment is associated with each stepwise in-

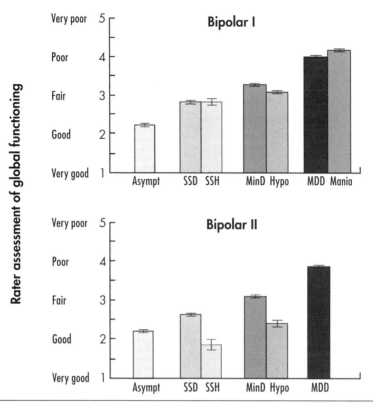

FIGURE 4–2.   Mean ratings of global psychosocial functioning by affective symptom severity category during long-term follow-up of Collaborative Depression Study patients with bipolar disorder.

Based on mixed model repeated measures analysis of functioning during months when the same subject was experiencing different categories of symptoms. Asympt = no symptoms of the affective episode (usual self); Hypo = hypomania threshold; Mania = manic episode threshold; MDD = major depressive episode threshold; MinD = minor depression/dysthymia threshold; SSD = subsyndromal depressive symptoms (below MinD threshold); SSH = subsyndromal hypomanic symptoms (below hypomania threshold).

crease or decrease in manic symptom severity. For those with bipolar II disorder, however, subsyndromal hypomanic symptoms are associated with slightly *enhanced* psychosocial function compared with the asymptomatic status, as reported by Akiskal and others (Akiskal 2002; Akiskal and Akiskal 1988; Akiskal et al. 2000; Jamison et al. 1980). During periods with symptoms at the hypomanic threshold, psychosocial functioning is about the same as when patients with bipolar II disorder are asymptomatic. The absence of significant impairment when patients with bipolar II disorder are experiencing mild or moderate symptoms in the manic spectrum may lead to low recognition and reporting of hypomanic or subhypomanic periods. Thus, time spent with these manic spectrum symptoms, and polarity shifts occurring at subsyndromal levels, may be substantially underreported for patients with bipolar II disorder in the CDS data presented here. Difficulty in recognizing hypomanic and subhypomanic periods may result in the even more serious problem of underdiagnosis of bipolar II disorder. Standard diagnostic procedures such as the Schedule for Affective Disorders and Schizophrenia (Endicott and Spitzer 1978) and the Structured Clinical Interview for DSM-IV Axis I Disorders (SCID; First et al. 1997), which do not adequately address subtle signs of bipolarity, may lead to misdiagnosis and inappropriate treatment of many patients with bipolar II disorder (Angst et al. 2003a; Benazzi and Akiskal 2001, 2003). Missed signs of underlying bipolarity were highlighted through analysis of 48 subjects who entered the CDS with a diagnosis of unipolar MDD but were later given the diagnosis of bipolar II disorder during follow-up (Akiskal et al. 1995). The strongest predictors of switching to a bipolar II diagnosis were patients' description of their "usual self," *during their intake MDE,* as characterized by heightened mood lability and by energy or activity. A modification of the SCID created by Benazzi and Akiskal (2003) is the current gold standard for identifying these and other signs of subtle bipolarity. A symptom checklist, the Hypomania Symptom Checklist (HCL-32), was developed by Angst et al. (2005) as a tool for identifying hypomanic states in patients with MDD. A revised version, the HCL-32-R_1 (Leao and Del Porto 2012), has been shown to be a sensitive self-report instrument that can supplement clinical interviews for identifying hypomanic and subthreshold hypomanic periods.

Clinical Importance of Bipolar II Disorder

Bipolar II disorder tends to be inappropriately regarded as the less serious of the two bipolar subtypes and, therefore, frequently treated with less vigor than bipolar I disorder. Our findings from the CDS show that patients with bipolar II disorder were symptomatic for half of the time (49.4% of weeks) during up to 30 years of follow-up—nearly as much as patients with bipolar I disorder, who were symptomatic during 53.2% of the weeks in their long-term course. Over a mean of 19 years of follow-up, they did not differ significantly from patients with bipolar I disorder in terms of the percentage of weeks with symptoms at the severity level of MDE or mania (11.8% vs. 14.4%) or in major affective episodes (23.8% vs. 29.2%). In our study comparing the episodic course of bipolar I and II disorders in the CDS (Judd et al. 2003a), we found that patients with bipolar II disorder had significantly longer intake episodes ($P < 0.001$). They also had marginally more episodes during the 10-year period after resolution of their intake episode ($P = 0.052$), including significantly more episodes of MDD and minor depression or dysthymia ($P < 0.001$ for both). As indicated previously in this chapter, mean overall level of psychosocial impairment during their long-term course also was the same as for bipolar I disorder; both bipolar groups experienced moderate or worse impairment during 30% of follow-up (Judd et al. 2008b).

Despite the evidence that bipolar II disorder is often an intensely chronic and recurrent disorder with a very high rate of depressive symptoms that are associated with significant psychosocial impairment, treatment of bipolar II disorder tends to be overlooked. We previously found that CDS patients with bipolar II disorder were prescribed somatic treatment significantly less often than were those with bipolar I disorder when they were experiencing depressive symptoms at the threshold for major depression (60.4% vs. 76.0%; $P = 0.003$) or minor depression or dysthymia (56.9% vs. 77.2%; $P < 0.001$) (Judd et al. 2003c). Prophylactic treatment for bipolar II disorder also was significantly lower, having been given during only 44.0% of weeks between affective episodes compared with 68.6% for those with bipolar I disorder ($P < 0.001$) (Judd et al. 2003a).

Data presented here clearly show that bipolar II disorder is *not* the lesser of the two bipolar subtypes but rather a serious, chronic disorder with high rates of impairing depressive symptoms and syndromes that warrant the same level of attention and treatment given to bipolar I disorder.

Importance of Asymptomatic Recovery From Major Affective Episodes

The presence of ongoing residual subsyndromal depressive symptoms following recovery from an MDE in patients with unipolar MDD, although meeting the consensus definition of "recovery," is associated with significantly faster episode relapse or recurrence when compared with full asymptomatic recovery (Judd et al. 1998b, 2000b). *Recovery* for our investigation of bipolar disorders (Judd et al. 2008a), as for unipolar MDD, followed the current consensus definition of being asymptomatic or having minimal residual affective symptoms for 8 or more consecutive weeks. We found (Figure 4–3) that those bipolar patients recovering from their intake MDE or manic episode with residual affective symptoms experienced a subsequent affective episode 3.4 times faster than did those who recovered to an asymptomatic state (median = 65 vs. 19 weeks, respectively; $P < 0.001$). Recovery with residual affective symptoms was associated with *major* affective episode relapse or recurrence more than five times faster than was asymptomatic recovery (median = 24 weeks vs. 123 weeks, respectively; $P < 0.001$). We also found that those whose recovery included residual affective symptoms had a significantly more chronic and severe future course of illness. Recovery status (asymptomatic vs. residual symptoms) proved to be the strongest correlate of time to major affective episode relapse or recurrence for the bipolar cohort ($P < 0.001$), followed by a history of three or more affective episodes before intake ($P = 0.007$). No other variable of the 13 examined was significantly associated with time to relapse or recurrence. We concluded that in bipolar disorder, the presence of residual symptoms after the resolution of a major affective episode indicates that the illness is still active and that the patient is at significant risk for rapid relapse or recurrence.

A panel of mood disorder experts has proposed a standardized set of definitions for recovery (Hirschfeld et al. 2007). These include *remission,* in which the patient has no or only minimal symptoms of the affective episode for 1 week, and *sustained remission,* in which this status is maintained for 8–12 consecutive weeks. Our finding that *recovery* with minimal residual affective symptoms predicts much faster episode relapse in unipolar (Judd et al. 1998b, 2000b) and bipolar (Judd et al. 2008a) patients, however, argues for a stricter definition of episode recovery based on resolution of *all* symptoms of the episode.

Berk et al. (2008) reanalyzed data from four treatment studies with a definition of *remission* based on achieving a Clinical Global Impression–Bipolar Version (CGI-BP) severity score of 1 ("normal, not at all ill"). These authors concluded that the stricter definition of remission (total absence of symptoms of the episode), although more difficult to attain, is more clinically meaningful. We fully agree and have been advocating this since 1998 (Judd et al. 1998b). The minimum time (number of consecutive weeks) at this status needed to define a stable state of recovery needs to be determined through empirical study and may be shorter than 8 weeks. With increasing knowledge about the mechanisms underlying mood disorder states and response to treatment, neurobiological measures of euthymia and a truly disease-free state are likely to be developed (Keller 2003). In the meantime, definitions of illness and recovery are based mainly on symptom status, and mounting evidence indicates that stable recovery from an affective episode is achieved only when the *asymptomatic* state is maintained for a sufficient time for the patient to be free of risk for relapse.

Summary of Findings Based on the Dimensional Paradigm of the Long-Term Course of Bipolar Disorders

Bipolar disorders (types I and II) are chronic, lifelong illnesses, with strong tendencies for relapse and recurrence of major and minor affective episodes.

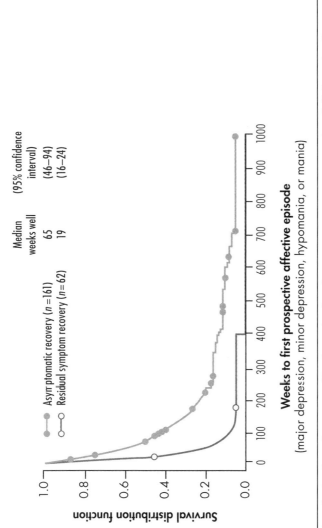

FIGURE 4–3. Survival analysis of weeks to any affective episode relapse or recurrence comparing Collaborative Depression Study patients with bipolar disorder (type I or II) who recovered from their intake major affective episode but have residual subsyndromal affective symptoms with the asymptomatic status.

Note. Wilcoxon χ^2 test of overall difference = 49.63; $P < 0.001$.

Syndromal affective episodes are interspersed with euthymic periods, during which subsyndromal symptoms are often present. The long-term symptomatic expression of bipolar disorders is dimensional in character, consisting of a continuum of depressive and manic or hypomanic symptom severity. Affective symptoms beneath the severity threshold of mania and major depression dominate the course of both bipolar I and bipolar II disorders, as do depressive episodes and symptoms. The long-term course of bipolar disorders is dynamic and changeable, with patients frequently moving between symptom polarity or severity categories. Psychosocial impairment is linked in a progressive stepwise fashion with each increase or decrease in depressive symptom severity in both bipolar disorders and with each increase or decrease in manic symptom severity in bipolar I disorder. When patients are without symptoms (asymptomatic), they return to good psychosocial function. Bipolar II disorder is not, as is often thought, the less serious of the two bipolar disorders but rather is an equally chronic and impairing, highly depressive disorder. Asymptomatic recovery from major affective episodes is associated with a significantly longer delay in episode relapse or recurrence, as well as a more benign future course of illness.

Clinical Implications

- Because of the chronic nature of bipolar disorders, it is imperative that health care systems provide ongoing monitoring by a clinician or case manager and care as needed over the long term.
- Patients, their families, and others who are part of the patients' support system should be given accurate information about the strong tendencies for episode relapse and recurrence; the early warning signs of an impending episode and the need to contact the clinician immediately; the need for strict adherence to recommended treatment regimens (both acute and extended); and the importance of bringing any treatment compliance problems to the attention of the clinician.
- The clinician should combine medication and adjunctive psychosocial interventions. A considerable body of evidence has been building to confirm the effectiveness of psychosocial intervention programs for improving both acute and long-term outcomes in bipolar illness. At a recent roundtable (Keck et al. 2007), experts in the field concluded that, as with other chronic mental disorders, the best strategy is an integrated approach that in-

cludes individualized programs of psychosocial intervention (such as cognitive-behavioral therapy, interpersonal and social rhythm therapy, and family therapy) together with acute and long-term medication regimens. Research results are promising and await further randomized controlled clinical trials that confirm or extend the early findings. In the meantime, it is recommended that integrated pharmacological and psychosocial therapies be used for bipolar I and II disorders, with the specific modalities selected and applied based on the most recent publications in this rapidly expanding area of research.

- Depressive episodes and symptoms should be treated with equal priority to manic episodes and symptoms. Collaborative Depression Study data provide strong evidence that the long-term course of bipolar I and II disorders is predominantly depressive and that every level of depressive symptom severity is associated with significantly greater psychosocial impairment.

- The clinician should treat bipolar II disorder with the same priority and rigor as bipolar I disorder. Results summarized here underscore the chronic and disabling nature of bipolar II disorder, together with the tendency to treat it less frequently than bipolar I disorder is treated at the same levels of affective symptom severity. Over the long-term course, bipolar II disorder is as impairing as bipolar I disorder because of its chronic and overwhelmingly depressive nature. Patients with bipolar II disorder need equal treatment priority and rigor to those with bipolar I disorder throughout their lifetime.

- All levels of depressive symptoms during bipolar illness and all levels of manic symptoms in bipolar I disorder must be treated because these are accompanied by significant psychosocial impairment.

- Affective episodes must be treated sufficiently to reach an asymptomatic state. The presence of ongoing residual affective symptoms following "recovery" from a major affective episode, even though the individual may meet consensus criteria for remission, is associated with early episode relapse and a worse future course of illness. The clinician's immediate goal is aggressive management of acute episodes with evidence-based treatments, but the ultimate goal should be attainment of the asymptomatic status long enough for a stable state of full episode recovery to be achieved.

- As with all chronic illnesses, the optimal goal for treatment of bipolar episodes, as for unipolar major depressive disorder, is to reduce chronicity, prevent exacerbations and recurrences, restore patients to their optimal level of psychosocial functioning, and maintain as symptom-free a state as possible throughout their lifetime.

References

Akiskal HS: Classification, diagnosis and boundaries of bipolar disorders, in Bipolar Disorder. Edited by Maj M, Akiskal HS, Lopez-Ibor JJ, et al. London, England, Wiley, 2002, pp 1–52

Akiskal HS, Akiskal K: Re-assessing the prevalence of bipolar disorders: clinical significance and artistic creativity. Psychiatrie et Psychobiologie 3:S29–S36, 1988

Akiskal HS, Benazzi F: Psychopathologic correlates of suicidal ideation in major depressive outpatients: is it all due to unrecognized (bipolar) depressive mixed states? Psychopathology 38:273–280, 2005

Akiskal HS, Maser JD, Zeller PJ, et al: Switching from 'unipolar' to bipolar II: an 11-year prospective study of clinical and temperamental predictors in 559 patients. Arch Gen Psychiatry 52:114–123, 1995

Akiskal HS, Bourgeois ML, Angst J, et al: Re-evaluating the prevalence of and diagnostic composition within the broad clinical spectrum of bipolar disorders. J Affect Disord 59 (suppl 1):S5–S30, 2000

American Psychiatric Association: Diagnostic and Statistical Manual of Mental Disorders, 3rd Edition. Washington, DC, American Psychiatric Association, 1980

American Psychiatric Association: Diagnostic and Statistical Manual of Mental Disorders, 4th Edition, Text Revision. Washington, DC, American Psychiatric Association, 2000

Angst J, Preisig M: Course of a clinical cohort of unipolar, bipolar and schizoaffective patients: results of a prospective study from 1959 to 1985. Schweiz Arch Neurol Psychiatr 146:5–16, 1995

Angst J, Gamma A, Benazzi F, et al: Toward a re-definition of subthreshold bipolarity: epidemiology and proposed criteria for bipolar-II, minor bipolar disorders and hypomania. J Affect Disord 73:133–146, 2003a

Angst J, Gamma A, Sellaro R, et al: Recurrence of bipolar disorders and major depression: a life-long perspective. Eur Arch Psychiatry Clin Neurosci 253:236–240, 2003b

Angst J, Adolfsson R, Benazzi F, et al: The HCL-32: towards a self-assessment tool for hypomanic symptoms in outpatients. J Affect Disord 88:217–233, 2005

Balázs J, Benazzi F, Rihmer Z, et al: The close link between suicide attempts and mixed (bipolar) depression: implications for suicide prevention. J Affect Disord 91:133–138, 2006

Benazzi F, Akiskal HS: Delineating bipolar II mixed states in the Ravenna-San Diego collaborative study: the relative prevalence and diagnostic significance of hypomanic features during major depressive episodes. J Affect Disord 67:115–122, 2001

Benazzi F, Akiskal HS: Refining the evaluation of bipolar II: beyond the strict SCID-CV guidelines for hypomania. J Affect Disord 73:33–38, 2003

Berk M, Ng F, Wang WV, et al: The empirical redefinition of the psychometric criteria for remission in bipolar disorder. J Affect Disord 106:153–158, 2008

Endicott J, Spitzer RL: A diagnostic interview: the Schedule for Affective Disorders and Schizophrenia. Arch Gen Psychiatry 35:837–844, 1978

First MC, Spitzer RL, Gibbon M, et al: Structured Clinical Interview for DSM-IV Axis I Disorders—Clinician Version (SCID-CV). Washington, DC, American Psychiatric Press, 1997

Frye MA, Helleman G, McElroy SL, et al: Correlates of treatment-emergent mania associated with antidepressant treatment in bipolar depression. Am J Psychiatry 166:164–172, 2009

Goldberg JF, Perlis RH, Ghaemi SN, et al: Adjunctive antidepressant use and symptomatic recovery among bipolar depressed patients with concomitant manic symptoms: findings from the STEP-BD. Am J Psychiatry 164:1348–1355, 2007

Goldberg JF, Perlis RH, Bowden CL, et al: Manic symptoms during depressive episodes in 1,380 patients with bipolar disorder: findings from the STEP-BD. Am J Psychiatry 166:173–181, 2009

Hawton K, Sutton L, Haw C, et al: Suicide and attempted suicide in bipolar disorder: a systematic review of risk factors. J Clin Psychiatry 66:693–704, 2005

Hirschfeld RM, Calabrese JR, Frye MA, et al: Defining the clinical course of bipolar disorder: response, remission, relapse, recurrence, and roughening. Psychopharmacol Bull 40:7–14, 2007

Jamison KR, Gerner RH, Hammen C, et al: Clouds and silver linings: positive experiences associated with primary affective disorders. Am J Psychiatry 137:198–202, 1980

Judd LL, Schettler PJ: The long-term course and clinical management of bipolar I and bipolar II disorders, in Bipolar Disorder: Clinical and Neurobiological Foundations. Edited by Yatham LN, Maj M. Chichester, West Sussex, UK, Wiley-Blackwell, 2010, pp 17–30

Judd LL, Akiskal HS, Maser JD, et al: A prospective 12-year study of subsyndromal and syndromal depressive symptoms in unipolar major depressive disorders. Arch Gen Psychiatry 55:694–700, 1998a

Judd LL, Akiskal HS, Maser JD, et al: Major depressive disorder: a prospective study of residual subthreshold depressive symptoms as a predictor of rapid relapse. J Affect Disord 50:97–108, 1998b

Judd LL, Akiskal HS, Zeller PJ, et al: Psychosocial disability during the long-term course of unipolar major depressive disorder. Arch Gen Psychiatry 57:375–380, 2000a

Judd LL, Paulus MP, Zeller PJ, et al: Does incomplete recovery from first lifetime major depressive episode herald a chronic course of illness? Am J Psychiatry 157:1501–1504, 2000b

Judd LL, Akiskal HS, Schettler PJ, et al: The long-term natural history of the weekly symptomatic status of bipolar I disorder. Arch Gen Psychiatry 59:530–537, 2002

Judd LL, Akiskal HS, Schettler PJ, et al: The comparative clinical phenotype and long-term longitudinal episode course of bipolar I and II: a clinical spectrum or distinct disorders? J Affect Disord 73:19–32, 2003a

Judd LL, Akiskal HS, Schettler PJ, et al: A prospective investigation of the natural history of the long-term weekly symptomatic status of bipolar II disorder. Arch Gen Psychiatry 60:261–269, 2003b

Judd LL, Schettler PJ, Akiskal HS, et al: Long-term symptomatic status of bipolar I vs. bipolar II disorders. Int J Neuropsychopharmacol 6:127–137, 2003c

Judd LL, Akiskal HS, Schettler PJ, et al: Psychosocial disability in the course of bipolar I and II disorders: a prospective, comparative, longitudinal study. Arch Gen Psychiatry 62:1322–1330, 2005

Judd LL, Schettler PJ, Akiskal HS, et al: Residual symptom recovery from major affective episodes in bipolar disorders and rapid episode relapse/recurrence. Arch Gen Psychiatry 65:386–394, 2008a

Judd LL, Schettler PJ, Solomon DA, et al: Psychosocial disability and work role function compared across the long-term course of bipolar I, bipolar II and unipolar major depressive disorders. J Affect Disord 108:49–58, 2008b

Judd LL, Schettler PJ, Akiskal H, et al: Prevalence and clinical significance of subsyndromal manic symptoms, including irritability and psychomotor agitation, during bipolar major depressive episodes. J Affect Disord 138:440–448, 2012

Katz MM, Klerman GL: Introduction: overview of the clinical studies program. Am J Psychiatry 136:49–51, 1979

Katz MM, Secunda SK, Hirschfeld RMA, et al: NIMH Clinical Research Branch Collaborative Program on the Psychobiology of Depression. Arch Gen Psychiatry 36:765–771, 1979

Keck PE Jr, McIntyre RS, Shelton RC: Bipolar depression: best practices for the outpatient. CNS Spectr 12 (suppl 20):1–14, 2007

Keller MB: Past, present, and future directions for defining optimal treatment outcome in depression: remission and beyond. JAMA 289:3152–3160, 2003

Keller M, Lavori P, Friedman B, et al: Longitudinal interval follow-up evaluation. Arch Gen Psychiatry 44:540–548, 1987

Leao IAT, Del Porto JA: Cross validation with the Mood Disorder Questionnaire (MDQ) of an instrument for the detection of hypomania in Brazil: the 32 item Hypomania Symptom Check-List, First Revision (HCL-32-R_1). J Affect Disord 140:215–221, 2012

Salvi V, Fagiolini A, Swartz HA, et al: The use of antidepressants in bipolar disorder. J Clin Psychiatry 69:1307–1318, 2008

Spitzer RL, Endicott J, Robins E: Research Diagnostic Criteria for a Selected Group of Functional Disorders, 3rd Edition. New York, New York Biometrics Research Division, New York State Psychiatric Institute, 1977

CHAPTER 5

Risk Factors for Suicide Attempts and Completions

William H. Coryell, M.D.

IT IS WELL ESTABLISHED that those who seek treatment for a mental disorder, whatever that disorder might be, are at increased risk for suicide attempts or completion. The likelihood of suicidal behavior ranges widely within this heterogeneous group, and clinicians rely on an array of demographic and clinical factors to judge the threat a given patient poses, in both the short term and the long term. This calculation shapes the steps a clinician takes to reduce risks, steps that range in intrusiveness from the simple provision of appropriate treatment for the presenting complaint and the monitoring of suicidal thoughts or plans, to increased surveillance by family members, to involuntary hospitalization.

Each approach to the study of these risk factors has its own advantages and disadvantages. Analyses of vital statistics provide large numbers with which to determine temporal trends in suicide rates by geographic region as well as differences in risks across age and sex groups. Such data, however, cannot identify how demographic risk factors operate differently across disorders. Among individuals with major depression, for instance, the male-to-female ratio for completed suicide appears to be far smaller than the 4:1 ratio typically found in the U.S. general population (Coryell and Young 2005).

Psychological autopsy studies have shaped our thinking about risk factors for suicide by showing that few suicides occur in the absence of a diagnosable mental disorder. The labor-intensive nature of these studies has limited sample sizes, and many have not included control groups. Those that did draw control subjects from community samples have been unable to compare, for instance, depressed individuals who committed suicide with those who did not. Moreover, bias from knowledge of whether an individual is a control or a victim must be assumed. Ascertainment of symptoms in such studies is also limited to what informants surmise from a victim's statements or behaviors and is limited in time to the period immediately preceding the decision to die.

Studies of completed suicide from clinically ascertained samples offer the opportunity to identify risk factors within a specified diagnostic group. The existence of diagnostically specific risk factors for suicide is not widely appreciated, although compelling evidence indicates marked differences across conditions. Murphy et al. (1992), for instance, found that the immediate antecedents of suicide in a group with alcoholism showed little overlap with those of a group with primary depressive disorder. Higher levels of education and good insight are among the most consistently identified risk factors for suicide within schizophrenia cohorts (Hor and Taylor 2010), but neither of these has emerged as a risk factor in studies of mood disorder. The study of diagnostically mixed groups selected on the basis of patient status or recent suicidal behavior may yield findings that do not apply well to individuals with a particular disorder.

Clinical cohort studies of risk factors for suicide can have retrospective or prospective designs. The former is much more easily executed but lacks systematic baseline assessment. Mention of a specific sign or symptom may be missing from the record because it was absent or because the interviewer failed to inquire about it. Retrospective assessment also cannot ensure standardized terminology because the various clinicians who produced the records may have differed in their use of descriptors such as "retarded," "psychotic," or "histrionic." Prospective approaches avoid both of these problems, but the low frequency of suicides within even high-risk samples necessitates large samples. Long periods of observation are also necessary to separate short-term risk factors from those that apply across subsequent episodes of illness. These factors, combined with the need for a thorough baseline assessment, result in the need for a sustained investment of effort. Not surprisingly, only a limited number of large-scale prospective studies are available.

Of course, the prospect of failed suicide attempts also concerns treating clinicians. Observations that ratios of unsuccessful to completed suicide attempts are as high as 45:1 in younger U.S. populations (Kessler et al. 2005) serve to underscore the reality that risk factors for these two events are likely to differ in important ways. Most long-term prospective studies have assessed only risk factors for completed suicide because they allowed for only one or a few widely spaced follow-up assessments, whereas an accurate evaluation of attempts requires shorter follow-up intervals. The assessment of separate risks for both suicide attempts and completions within the same study is preferable because such a distinction allows for far firmer conclusions about the difference than do comparisons of the two sets of risk factors across studies.

The Collaborative Depression Study (CDS) cohort of 936 subjects with Research Diagnostic Criteria major depressive disorder, schizoaffective disorder, or manic disorder included 311 (33.2%) who described on intake at least one prior suicide attempt, 140 (15.0%) who described multiple previous attempts, and 178 (19.0%) who described at least one attempt that had intent rated as "serious" or medical lethality risk rated as "moderate or worse" (Fiedorowicz et al. 2009). After thorough baseline evaluation, individuals were reinterviewed at intervals of 6 months to a year. During a median follow-up of 19 years, the 909 participants with at least one follow-up assessment included 279 (30.7%) with at least one suicide attempt, 162 (17.8%) with multiple attempts, 176 (19.4%) with at least one attempt meeting the previously described definition of "serious" (Fiedorowicz et al. 2009), and 40 (4.4%) who completed suicide. The CDS has generated a data set uniquely suited to identifying risk factors for suicidal completions and suicide attempts among treatment-seeking individuals with mood disorders.

Clinical Risk Factors for Suicide Attempts

Symptoms and Temperament

Maser et al. (2002) tested an extensive array of clinical and historical variables as well as measures of temperament as risk factors for serious suicide attempts, both in the short term (1 year or less) and in the long term. *Serious* attempts had both a definite intent and a medical outcome that posed at least a moderate threat to life. A factor analysis of the 436 items in the baseline personality self-assessment battery generated 10 factors that differentiated among those who made serious attempts, those who completed suicide, and a comparison group of subjects with no suicidal behavior during follow-up. Suicide in affective disorders is discussed further in Chapter 15 ("Impact of Anxiety Severity on Mood Disorders").

Features that carried the highest relative risks for serious suicide attempts in both the short and the long term were a history of suicide attempt(s) with definite intent and substance abuse within the index episode. Relative risk values generally were larger for attempts that occurred in the first year of follow-up (Table 5–1). After the first year of follow-up, however, derived temperament predictors were much more consistent risk factors for serious suicide attempts and can therefore serve as a valuable complement to clinical predictors in assessing long-term risk. Significant predictors of serious suicide attempts after 1 year included high scores for shyness, brooding, dependence, rejection sensitivity, and impulsivity and low scores for sanguinity, assertiveness, and directed energy.

Of particular note, a history of serious suicide attempt(s) was strongly predictive of subsequent attempts in both the short and the long term, and this was so whether the prior attempt had occurred in the index episode or in a previous one. Clark et al. (1989) had shown this in an earlier CDS analysis that had focused on the question of whether the importance of a past attempt diminished as that attempt became more remote. They concluded that it did not; an attempt made years earlier was as important as a much more recent one in indicating an elevated risk for a future attempt.

The preceding analyses tested baseline measures as predictors of the first serious suicide attempt during follow-up. Individuals may have had multiple attempts over a lengthy observation period, and baseline measures such as age, comorbidity, symptom severity, and history of suicide attempts to that point will change over time. A subsequent analysis used a mixed-effect, grouped-time survival analysis to assess risk factors for suicidal behavior across 4,204 prospectively observed mood episodes (Fiedorowicz et al. 2009). Older age emerged as significantly protective. With age at episode onset included as a continuous covariate, hopelessness (hazard ratio=3.00) and substance abuse (hazard ratio=2.3) were significant risk factors, whereas being male, being unmarried, and a history of suicide attempts were not. The fact that most individuals with any prospectively observed attempt made multiple attempts during follow-up may have diminished the importance of a history of attempts before intake as a risk factor for any given attempt during follow-up.

Polarity

Earlier retrospective studies (Dunner et al. 1976; Kupfer et al. 1988) and at least one prospective study (Tondo et al. 2007) described higher rates of suicide attempts among individuals with bipolar illness than among those with unipolar illness. When age at first lifetime onset was controlled in a logistic regression, CDS data showed bipolar subjects to have a 30% higher likelihood of prior serious suicide attempts (Fiedorowicz et al. 2009). Prospectively as well, those with bipolar disorder had significantly higher rates of any attempt, multiple attempts, and serious attempts. However, across multiple prospectively observed mood episodes, polarity was not associated with risk for suicidal behavior after the study controlled for age at episode onset.

Rapid cycling, as defined by DSM-IV-TR (American Psychiatric Association 2000), occurs almost exclusively among individuals with bipolar disorder and appears to be a potent risk factor for suicide attempts. CDS subjects observed

TABLE 5–1. Short- and long-term risks for serious suicide attempts: significant intake symptoms and diagnostic variables

First year		Beyond first year	
Risk factor	**RR**	**Risk factor**	**RR**
Drug abuse in index episode	2.9	Any past suicide attempt with definite intent	2.5
Any past suicide attempt with definite intent	2.5	Alcohol abuse in index episode	2.0
Alcoholism or substance use disorder at index	2.4	Suicidal tendencies in index episode	1.7
Alcohol abuse in index episode	2.1	Not homemaker, student, or full-time worker for year prior to index episode	1.5
Ever alcohol or substance use disorder	2.1	≥4 lifetime episodes	1.4
Suicidal tendencies in index episode	1.7	Dissatisfied with life other than education or occupation	1.3
Dissatisfied with life other than education or occupation	1.4	Psychic anxiety in index episode	1.3
Hopelessness in index episode	1.3	Indecisiveness in index episode	1.3

Note. Analysis was limited to variables present in at least 10% of overall sample. Risk factors shown in the table are those with a significant contrast to the control group with no suicidal behavior during follow-up (after co-varying for age and gender) and a RR of 1.3 or higher.
RR=relative risk, the ratio of the percentage of the target group (patients with short- or long-term serious suicide attempts) who have the risk factor to the percentage within the control group (patients with no suicidal behavior of any degree of severity during follow-up).
Source. Maser et al. 2002.

to have a rapid-cycling course during their first year of follow-up were more than twice as likely to have histories of serious suicide attempts before study intake and were more than twice as likely to make such attempts during follow-up (Coryell et al. 2003).

Treatment

Although participation in the CDS did not influence treatment, follow-up assessments included a week-to-week account of all psychiatric medicine prescribed. This record afforded opportunities to assess potentially causal relations between changes in psychopathology and changes in the treatment levels of specific drug classes. Because dynamic clinical variables such as current symptom severity can drive both treatment level and outcomes of interest such as later symptom level and suicidal behaviors, CDS authors have used a statistical technique, *propensity analysis*, that adjusts for such variables. Because anecdotal reports had, at the time, chiefly implicated fluoxetine as a possible cause of increased suicidal behaviors, the first analysis focused on whether fluoxetine use changed risks for suicidal behavior (Leon et al. 1999). CDS data showed that both the severity of psychopathology and the cumulative number of suicide attempts increased the risk for subsequent attempts, whereas the use of fluoxetine and other antidepressants resulted in statistically insignificant reductions in the likelihood of suicidal behavior. The passage of time afforded a much longer observation period and a greater number of events, which allowed a similar analysis 12 years later that showed a significant 20% reduction in suicidal behaviors with ongoing antidepressant use (Leon et al. 2011).

Clinical Risk Factors for Completed Suicides

The two earliest CDS analyses of risk factors for completed suicide took different approaches. The first used data from an average of 4 years of follow-up to test 121 demographic, diagnostic, symptom-based, and historic variables (Fawcett et al. 1987) that differentiated 25 patients who committed suicide from 929 who did not. Among features present in at least 10% of the sample tested as having been present or absent, mood cycling within the index episode was most strongly associated with suicide, half (52%) of which occurred during the first year after entry into the study. When features were treated as continuous measures to take severity into account, hopelessness and anhedonia during the intake episode conveyed the highest risk.

With the next analysis, the total number of suicides had increased from 25 to 32 (Fawcett et al. 1990). The authors limited analysis to 46 items chosen as potential risk factors, first for suicides that occurred within the first year of follow-up and then for those that occurred later. Severe anhedonia, global insomnia, severe psychic anxiety, panic attacks, alcohol abuse, and diminished concentration were significant short-term predictors, whereas severe hopelessness, suicidal ideation, and a history of suicide attempts were risk factors for later suicide.

Twelve years later and with an additional four suicides, Maser et al. (2002) conducted a test of all variables that had been identified as potential predictors in earlier CDS analyses. They again separated short-term ($n=11$) and long-term

(n=25) suicide completers. All features were treated as dichotomies, and all tests covaried for age and sex. Also tested were 19 features derived from 436 items contained in the CDS intake personality battery. The highest relative risk factor for short-term suicide was a delusion of thought insertion during the index episode (Table 5–2). Otherwise, substance abuse figured prominently, as did having a cycling or mixed polarity episode at intake, experiencing panic attacks or psychic anxiety during the episode, or having no children younger than 18 years living in the home. A history of any suicide attempt with definite intent was one of the highest long-term risk factors for completed suicide. This underscores earlier findings that even remote attempts indicate a traitlike proneness to such behavior. Another risk factor for long-term suicide, the absence of a role of homemaker, student, or employee during the year before intake, is likely a proxy for chronic isolation and disability, as may be the item "dissatisfaction with life other than education or occupation." Additional risk factors for long-term suicide included drug abuse, delusions or hallucinations, suicidal tendencies, indecisiveness, and hopelessness in the index episode.

Fewer temperament measures were significantly associated with suicide completions, whether short-term (5) or long-term (8), than were associated with suicide attempts (10 and 19, respectively), as would be expected given the very large difference in the number of subjects with suicide attempts (n=84) compared with those with suicide completions (n=36). As with attempts, temperament factors were much more strongly related to long-term than to short-term suicides. Among the more prominent long-term predictors were shyness and impulsivity. Sanguinity was protective.

In an effort to determine which course variables ascertained during follow-up were associated with completed suicide, 29 individuals who committed suicide were matched to those who did not by age, sex, lifetime drug or alcohol abuse, polarity, and time since last interview (Coryell et al. 2002). Suicide was associated with having more weeks during follow-up with any affective morbidity. The tendency toward greater affective illness morbidity among those who completed suicide was apparent in each year of follow-up and in each of the final 6 months prior to suicide. Surprisingly, those who completed suicide showed no tendency as a group to experience steadily worsening morbidity over time. Previous suicide attempts of high intent or lethality were strongly associated with eventual suicide whether they had occurred during follow-up, in the index episode before study intake, or in a previous episode. With all periods considered together, only one (3.4%) of the patients who completed suicide lacked a history of attempts, whereas more than a third of the matched control subjects (37.9%) had no prior serious attempt. Contrary to expectation, the predictive importance of a history of a high intent attempt was somewhat larger for attempts that had occurred prior to the index episode than for those that had occurred in the index episode or during follow-up.

TABLE 5–2. Short- and long-term risk factors for completed suicide: significant intake symptoms and diagnostic variables

First year		Beyond first year	
Risk factor	**RR**	**Risk factor**	**RR**
Delusions of thought insertion in index episode	22.8	Not homemaker, student, or full-time worker for year prior to index episode	3.2
Alcoholism or substance use disorder at index	3.5	Any past suicide attempt with definite intent	2.5
Cycling or mixed index affective episode	2.3	Drug abuse in index episode	2.0
Ever alcoholism or substance use disorder	2.1	Delusions or hallucinations in index episode	1.9
Panic attack in index episode	1.8	Suicidal tendencies in index episode	1.6
Psychic anxiety in index episode	1.8	Dissatisfied with life other than education or occupation	1.5
No children age 18 or younger in home	1.6	Indecisiveness in index episode	1.5
		Hopelessness in index episode	1.3

Note. Analysis was limited to variables present in at least 10% of overall sample. Risk factors shown in the table are those with a significant contrast to the control group with no suicidal behavior during follow-up (after covarying for age and gender) and a RR of 1.3 or higher.

RR = relative risk, the ratio of the percentage of the target group (patients with short- or long-term completed suicides) who have the risk factor to the percentage within the control group (patients with no suicidal behavior of any degree of severity during follow-up).

Source. Maser et al. 2002.

Biological Risk Factors for Suicide Attempts and Completions

Subject recruitment into the CDS coincided with a period when the dexamethasone suppression test (DST) was being widely researched as a possible laboratory test for melancholia. Because the Iowa Center was one of the departments then actively investigating the DST as a diagnostic tool for mood disorder, 77 of the CDS probands also had been recruited into a study to test the role of DST in diagnostic subtyping. Because earlier research that used measures of urinary free cortisol (Bunney and Fawcett 1965), adrenal weight (Dorovini-Zis and Zis 1987; Szigethy et al. 1994), and adrenal volume (Willenberg et al. 1998) had identified hypothalamic-pituitary-adrenal (HPA) axis hyperactivity as a risk factor for suicide, the Iowa investigators compared the CDS patients whose positive DST results had indicated HPA axis hyperactivity with those who had had normal DST results (Coryell 1990). Although these two groups did not differ in terms of overall likelihood of suicide attempts during follow-up, nonsuppressors were significantly more likely to have made attempts that were of high intent, and those with normal results were somewhat more likely to have made attempts that were of low intent.

Group differences in the proportions with completed suicide were more striking (Coryell and Schlesser 2001). Survival estimates indicated an eventual risk for suicide of 26.8% for the 32 subjects who had been DST nonsuppressors, but only 2.9% for those who had had normal results. Notably, survival curves for time to suicide in the two groups continued to diverge many years after the baseline testing. This indicated that HPA axis hyperactivity conveyed an increased risk for completed suicide that extended well beyond the index depressive episode.

A substantial literature linking low serum cholesterol concentrations to risks for both suicide attempts and suicide completions led the Iowa investigators to test this value as a risk factor (Coryell and Schlesser 2007). In a model with age, a cholesterol concentration below the group median was significantly associated with later suicide. Moreover, because DST results were uncorrelated with cholesterol concentrations, the predictive effects of the two tests were additive. Three (30.0%) of the 10 who had had both below-median cholesterol concentrations and an abnormal DST result died by suicide, but none of the 30 with higher cholesterol concentrations and a normal DST result did so. Groups with other value combinations had intermediate risks.

Subjects with low cholesterol concentrations also were more likely to have had suicide attempts, both before and during their index episodes (Fiedorowicz and Coryell 2007). Surprisingly, cholesterol concentrations were not predictive of suicide attempts during follow-up, and among younger subjects, low concentrations were associated, instead, with fewer attempts.

Mann and Currier (2007) described nine studies that tracked completed suicide in cohorts with major depression, relative to baseline DST results. Of these, seven described substantially higher rates among those with baseline evidence of HPA axis hyperactivity. The very substantial data linking total cholesterol level with suicide risk (Coryell and Schlesser 2007) and the likelihood that this may constitute a clinically assessable measure of low serotonin functioning (Muldoon et al. 1992) render the combined use of this measure with measures of HPA axis activity a potentially powerful predictor of long-term risk for completed suicide.

Clinical Implications

- A history of a suicide attempt, however remote, is a potent risk factor for future attempts.
- A history of a suicide attempt of high intent, however remote, is a potent risk factor for completed suicide.
- Substance abuse is a risk factor for both suicide attempts and completions, both short- and long-term.
- Certain measures of temperament are relatively strong predictors of long-term risks for suicidal behaviors.
- Antidepressant use decreases the risk of suicidal behavior.

References

American Psychiatric Association: Diagnostic and Statistical Manual of Mental Disorders, 4th Edition, Text Revision. Washington, DC, American Psychiatric Association, 2000

Bunney WE Jr, Fawcett JA: Possibility of a biochemical test for suicidal potential: an analysis of endocrine findings prior to three suicides. Arch Gen Psychiatry 13:232–239, 1965

Clark DC, Gibbons RD, Fawcett J, et al: What is the mechanism by which suicide attempts predispose to later suicide attempts? A mathematical model. J Abnorm Psychol 98:42–49, 1989

Coryell W: DST abnormality as a predictor of course in major depression. J Affect Disord 19:163–169, 1990

Coryell W, Schlesser M: The dexamethasone suppression test and suicide prediction. Am J Psychiatry 158:748–753, 2001

Coryell W, Schlesser M: Combined biological tests for suicide prediction. Psychiatry Res 150:187–191, 2007

Coryell W, Young EA: Clinical predictors of suicide in primary major depressive disorder. J Clin Psychiatry 66:412–417, 2005

Coryell W, Haley J, Endicott J, et al: The prospectively observed course of illness among depressed patients who commit suicide. Acta Psychiatr Scand 105:218–223, 2002

Coryell W, Solomon D, Turvey C, et al: The long-term course of rapid-cycling bipolar disorder. Arch Gen Psychiatry 60:914–920, 2003

Dorovini-Zis K, Zis AP: Increased adrenal weight in victims of violent suicide. Am J Psychiatry 144:1214–1215, 1987

Dunner DL, Gershon ES, Goodwin FK: Heritable factors in the severity of affective illness. Biol Psychiatry 11:31–42, 1976

Fawcett J, Scheftner W, Clark D, et al: Clinical predictors of suicide in patients with major affective disorders: a controlled prospective study. Am J Psychiatry 144:35–40, 1987

Fawcett J, Scheftner WA, Fogg L, et al: Time-related predictors of suicide in major affective disorder. Am J Psychiatry 147:1189–1194, 1990

Fiedorowicz JG, Coryell WH: Cholesterol and suicide attempts: a prospective study of depressed inpatients. Psychiatry Res 152:11–20, 2007

Fiedorowicz JG, Leon AC, Keller MB, et al: Do risk factors for suicidal behavior differ by affective disorder polarity? Psychol Med 39:763–771, 2009

Hor K, Taylor M: Suicide and schizophrenia: a systematic review of rates and risk factors. J Psychopharmacol 24 (4 suppl):81–90, 2010

Kessler RC, Berglund P, Borges G, et al: Trends in suicide ideation, plans, gestures, and attempts in the United States, 1990–1992 to 2001–2003. JAMA 293:2487–2495, 2005

Kupfer DJ, Carpenter LL, Frank E: Is bipolar II a unique disorder? Compr Psychiatry 29:228–236, 1988

Leon AC, Keller MB, Warshaw MG, et al: Prospective study of fluoxetine treatment and suicidal behavior in affectively ill subjects. Am J Psychiatry 156:195–201, 1999

Leon AC, Solomon DA, Li C, et al: Antidepressants and risks of suicide and suicide attempts: a 27-year observational study. J Clin Psychiatry 72:580–586, 2011

Mann JJ, Currier D: A review of prospective studies of biologic predictors of suicidal behavior in mood disorders. Arch Suicide Res 11:3–16, 2007

Maser JD, Akiskal HS, Schettler P, et al: Can temperament identify affectively ill patients who engage in lethal or near-lethal suicidal behavior? A 14-year prospective study. Suicide Life Threat Behav 32:10–32, 2002

Muldoon MF, Kaplan JR, Manuck SB, et al: Effects of a low-fat diet on brain serotonergic responsivity in cynomolgus monkeys. Biol Psychiatry 31:739–742, 1992

Murphy GE, Wetzel RD, Robins E, et al: Multiple risk factors predict suicide in alcoholism. Arch Gen Psychiatry 49:459–463, 1992

Szigethy E, Conwell Y, Forbes NT, et al: Adrenal weight and morphology in victims of completed suicide. Biol Psychiatry 36:374–380, 1994

Tondo L, Lepri B, Baldessarini RJ: Suicidal risks among 2826 Sardinian major affective disorder patients. Acta Psychiatr Scand 116:419–428, 2007

Willenberg HS, Bornstein SR, Dumser T, et al: Morphological changes in adrenals from victims of suicide in relation to altered apoptosis. Endocr Res 24:963–967, 1998

CHAPTER 6

Psychotic Features in Major Depressive and Manic Episodes

William H. Coryell, M.D.

THE CONCURRENCE of psychotic features with major affective syndromes raises two important questions. The first concerns the fundamental distinction between major mood disorders and schizophrenia and whether the coexisting psychotic features in a given case indicate by their nature that outcome and treatment response are likely to be consistent with schizophrenia or with a mood disorder. The frequency with which this question arises in clinical settings has resulted in a large but inconclusive literature around the concept of schizoaffective disorder. The many shifts in how the term has been defined have reflected the uncertainty of its meaning and make summaries of this literature difficult.

The second question presumes that an affective disorder is present but asks whether the presence of psychotic features is predictive of the future course of illness and is relevant to the optimal treatments for it. Interest in these questions began with observations that individuals with psychotic depression were less likely to recover while taking tricyclic antidepressants than those with nonpsychotic depression (Friedman et al. 1961; Glassman et al. 1975; Hordern et al. 1963). Because psychotic features did not appear to have importance for the acute or prophylactic effects of lithium, the studies that address the significance of psychotic features within depressive episodes far outnumber those that consider the importance of psychotic features within manic syndromes.

83

Data from the Collaborative Depression Study (CDS) are particularly well suited to address these two questions. In addition to the obvious strengths of a lengthy follow-up with high surveillance intensity, the use of the Schedule for Affective Disorders and Schizophrenia (Endicott and Spitzer 1978) to assess baseline phenomenology provides coverage of psychotic features that is exceptional in scope. The Research Diagnostic Criteria (RDC; Spitzer et al. 1978) definition of schizoaffective disorder was likewise usefully broad in that it required only that a full major depressive or manic syndrome be accompanied by one feature from a specified list of first-rank psychotic symptoms. It then provided for alternative subtypes, one based on the nature and timing of psychotic and affective symptoms and the other on episode duration. In the former, individuals with mainly schizophrenic schizoaffective disorder described either of two symptom sequences: 1) a period of a week or more during which mood-incongruent psychotic features were present without prominent manic or depressive symptoms and 2) the presence, prior to the onset of affective features, of social withdrawal, impairment in occupational functioning, eccentric behavior, emotional blunting, or unusual thoughts or perceptual experiences. Those who lacked these features had mainly affective schizoaffective disorder. The subtype based on chronicity used "acute," "subacute," "subchronic," and "chronic" to distinguish groups on the basis of episode duration and the completeness of recovery from earlier episodes.

Significance of Psychotic Features Generally

Psychotic Features in Major Depression

Early CDS reports focused on the effect of psychotic features on the course that preceded intake, on the subsequent persistence of depressive symptoms, and on the levels of psychosocial functioning in the first several years of follow-up. Results showed that subjects with psychotic depression were, in comparison to those with nonpsychotic major depression, more often incapacitated at the time of intake and more impaired in various psychosocial spheres, both immediately before intake and during their best and worst periods in the 5 years preceding intake (Coryell et al. 1987a). Those with psychotic features also experienced a nonsignificantly greater persistence of depressive symptoms in the first 6 months (Coryell et al. 1984). At 2 years, however, patients with baseline psychotic features were no less likely to have recovered (Coryell et al. 1984), and group differences in psychosocial adjustment had narrowed considerably or had disappeared (Coryell et al. 1987a).

Initial CDS comparisons of psychotic and nonpsychotic depression adhered to RDC conventions, in which individuals with first-rank symptoms were designated schizoaffective and thus were not included in the psychotic depression grouping. As a way of providing findings comparable to those that used DSM-III-R (American Psychiatric Association 1987) definitions, the psychotic depression grouping was modified to include all who had delusions or hallucinations but who did not meet RDC for the mainly schizophrenic subtype. The later grouping was equivalent to the relatively narrow DSM-IV (American Psychiatric Association 1994) definition of schizoaffective disorder. Thus, many who had schizoaffective disorder according to the RDC had a mood disorder with mood-incongruent psychotic features in the DSM-III (American Psychiatric Association 1980) system (Coryell et al. 1985). This shift in boundaries produced much larger outcome differences between psychotic and nonpsychotic groups such that the psychotic depression group experienced significantly more weeks in depressive episodes in each of the first 10 years of follow-up (Coryell et al. 1996). Group differences in levels of psychosocial impairment were now significant at 5 and 10 years.

The negative effect of baseline psychotic features on future depressive morbidity raised the possibility that psychotic features were simply an indicator of severity and that severity itself was the more fundamental correlate of long-term morbidity. How such severity should best be measured is uncertain, but a comparison of psychotic and nonpsychotic groups by the severity ratings of individual symptoms clearly showed higher symptom intensities in the psychotic group (Coryell et al. 1985). This was particularly evident for the depressive symptoms that constituted the criteria for major depression or for the endogenous subtype. Seven (41.2%) of the 17 core symptoms, but only 2 of the 13 (15.4%) noncriteria depressive symptoms, were significantly more severe in the psychotic group. In none of the 30 symptom comparisons was severity significantly greater in the nonpsychotic group.

Family study analyses provided evidence that psychotic features signify something more than a higher level of symptom severity (Endicott et al. 1986). Of the 40 probands who met RDC for psychotic major depressive disorder and who also had first-degree relatives directly interviewed by raters blind to proband diagnosis, 10% had at least one relative with a history of psychotic major depression, and another 5% had a relative with RDC schizoaffective disorder. Both values were significantly higher than the corresponding proportions of 2.6% and 0.4% for the probands with nonpsychotic major depressive disorder.

The *diagnostic stability* of a subtype refers to the consistency with which it manifests across subsequent episodes and is considered an indicator of diagnostic validity (Coryell et al. 1994). The psychotic subtype had modest diagnostic stability that, nevertheless, clearly exceeded that for the agitated/retarded and endogenous subtypes. More than a quarter (28.2%) of those who showed psychotic features in their index episode were again psychotic during their next relapse. In contrast, only 6 of 353 (1.7%) of those with a nonpsychotic index episode had psychotic features during their first relapse. For the index to first relapse pair, the κ value was 0.35 ($P<0.001$) and declined to 0.21 ($P=0.03$) for the index to fourth relapse pair. In contrast, for the agitated/retarded subtype, the κ value decreased from 0.16 ($P<0.001$) for the index to the first relapse pair to 0.02 (nonsignificant) for the index to the forth relapse pair. The corresponding κ values for the endogenous subtype were 0.17 ($P=0.0003$) and 0.12 (nonsignificant).

Although some reports found that psychotic depression was associated with higher rates of completed suicide or serious attempts (Roose et al. 1983), others have not (Coryell and Tsuang 1982). In the CDS sample, psychotic features were not among the baseline clinical features associated with either serious suicide attempts or suicide completions (Coryell et al. 2001; Maser et al. 2002).

Psychotic Features and Manic Episodes

A more recent CDS report compared individuals who had experienced psychotic features as a part of an index manic episode (other than those with mainly schizophrenic subtype of RDC schizoaffective disorder) with individuals whose index manic episode had lacked psychotic features. The former experienced fewer symptom-free weeks in each of the 15 years of follow-up, and the group differences did not lessen over time (Coryell et al. 2001). The psychotic group had more psychosocial impairment, and differences from the nonpsychotic group in these measures were greater at 10 years than they were at 5 years and were significant at both times. The prognostic significance of psychotic features in manic syndromes was therefore quite similar to their importance in depressive syndromes (Coryell et al. 1996). The presence of psychotic features within manic episodes, however, was not as predictive of future psychotic mania as the presence of psychotic features within major depressive episodes was predictive of future psychotic depression. A third (36.1%) of individuals with an index episode of psychotic mania had psychotic features in their next manic episode, but 18.9% of those whose index mania was nonpsychotic had psychotic features with their next mania (κ=0.18; $P=0.026$) (Coryell et al. 2001).

Schizoaffective Depression

A review of CDS findings on schizoaffective depression must begin with a review of how the RDC definition differs from the current DSM definition. The RDC definition is much broader and includes all individuals with any first-rank symptom such as delusions of thought broadcasting or passivity, even when such symptoms occur only during a major depressive or manic episode. The DSM-IV-TR (American Psychiatric Association 2000) definition of schizoaffective disorder requires that, at some time during the illness, delusions or hallucinations be present for at least 2 weeks in the absence of prominent mood symptoms. Many individuals with RDC schizoaffective disorder therefore have symptoms that meet DSM-IV-TR criteria for major depression or mania with mood-incongruent psychotic features.

The earliest CDS reports did not subtype schizoaffective depression and found that outcomes for subjects with this label were consistently, although not significantly, worse than those for patients with either RDC psychotic depression or nonpsychotic major depression (Coryell et al. 1984). A later report used 5 years of observations to compare 73 individuals with psychotic depression with 30 individuals who began the study with RDC schizoaffective depression (Coryell et al. 1990a). Poorer outcomes in the latter group were reflected in significantly higher rates of rehospitalization, greater proportions of follow-up with depressive syndromes, lower likelihood of recovery from the index episode, and higher likelihood of psychotic features sustained in the final 6 months of follow-up.

The subtyping of schizoaffective disorder indicates considerable prognostic heterogeneity (Coryell et al. 1987b). The distinction between mainly schizophrenic and mainly affective groups was important for those whose disorder was not also chronic (continuously ill for 2 or more years). In turn, the distinction between chronic and nonchronic was important only within the mainly affective group. Those who were neither chronically ill nor mainly schizophrenic were three times more likely to recover than were those who were either chronically ill or mainly schizophrenic.

Three types of evidence from CDS data indicate that a subset of individuals with RDC schizoaffective disorder may have a schizophrenia diathesis. First, family study data (Endicott et al. 1986) showed that the relatives of probands with schizoaffective disorder were more likely to have an unspecified functional psychosis than were the relatives of probands with RDC psychotic depression ($P = 0.016$). Second, individuals who entered the study with schizoaffective disorder were twice as likely to have psychotic features present throughout the final 6 months of the first 5-year follow-up period as were subjects who began with psychotic major depression ($P = 0.032$) (Coryell et al. 1990a). Among the baseline measures associated with a chronically psychotic outcome, a "history of mood-incongruent psychotic features to the relative exclusion of depressive symptoms" emerged as the most important predictor in a regression analysis. Third, a comparison of subjects with major depression whose psychotic features were "completely consistent with depressed mood" with subjects whose psychotic features "were not at all consistent with depressed mood" showed that the severity of five criteria for depressive symptoms was significantly higher in the mood-congruent group, whereas no symptoms were more severe in the mood-incongruent groups (Coryell et al.

1985). Thus, those with mood-congruent features showed a symptom pattern indicative of a severe depressive episode.

Schizoaffective Mania

An examination of the first 5 years of follow-up for 14 patients who began in episodes of schizoaffective mania and 56 who began with psychotic mania showed poorer outcomes in the former group, who spent significantly more weeks in hospital and had lower mean Global Assessment Scale (GAS) scores at the end of each 6-month period (Coryell et al. 1990b). The smaller numbers with schizoaffective mania did not permit an exploration of heterogeneity equivalent to that done for schizoaffective depression. When subjects with schizoaffective mania and psychotic mania were pooled, however, a regression analysis of those baseline features associated with a chronically psychotic outcome found that the most important predictors were a history of any formal thought disorder in the absence of prominent manic symptoms ($P=0.0002$), a loosening of associations at intake ($P=0.0056$), and a low GAS score at intake ($P=0.0134$). Thus, for both depressive and manic syndromes accompanied by various psychotic features, the most important predictor of chronic psychosis 5 years later was a history of mood-incongruent psychotic features in the absence of, or to the relative inclusion of, the corresponding mood syndrome.

Clinical Implications

- The presence of psychotic features within both major depressive and manic episodes portends greater long-term morbidity manifested in a greater percentage of time in mood disorder episodes.
- Psychotic features that accompany major depressive episodes increase the eventual risk of a chronic psychosis, but those that accompany manic episodes do not.
- Psychotic depression is characterized by greater severity of those symptoms that constitute the criteria for major depression or the melancholic subtype of major depression.
- For both psychotic depression and psychotic mania, one of the most important predictors of a chronically psychotic outcome is a history of mood-incongruent psychotic features that have occurred at some point in the absence of or to the relative exclusion of a corresponding mood syndrome.

References

American Psychiatric Association: Diagnostic and Statistical Manual of Mental Disorders, 3rd Edition. Washington, DC, American Psychiatric Association, 1980

American Psychiatric Association: Diagnostic and Statistical Manual of Mental Disorders, 3rd Edition, Revised. Washington, DC, American Psychiatric Association, 1987

American Psychiatric Association: Diagnostic and Statistical Manual of Mental Disorders, 4th Edition. Washington, DC, American Psychiatric Association, 1994

American Psychiatric Association: Diagnostic and Statistical Manual of Mental Disorders, 4th Edition, Text Revision. Washington, DC, American Psychiatric Association, 2000

Coryell W, Tsuang MT: Primary unipolar depression and the prognostic importance of delusions. Arch Gen Psychiatry 30:1181–1184, 1982

Coryell W, Lavori P, Endicott J, et al: Outcome in schizoaffective, psychotic, and nonpsychotic depression: course during a six- to 24-month follow-up. Arch Gen Psychiatry 41:787–791, 1984

Coryell W, Endicott J, Keller M, et al: Phenomenology and family history in DSM-III psychotic depression. J Affect Disord 9:13–18, 1985

Coryell W, Endicott J, Keller M: The importance of psychotic features to major depression: course and outcome during a 2-year follow-up. Acta Psychiatr Scand 75:78–85, 1987a

Coryell W, Grove W, VanEerdewegh M, et al: Outcome in RDC schizoaffective depression: the importance of diagnostic subtyping. J Affect Disord 12:47–56, 1987b

Coryell W, Keller M, Lavori P, et al: Affective syndromes, psychotic features, and prognosis, I: depression. Arch Gen Psychiatry 47:651–657, 1990a

Coryell W, Keller M, Lavori P, et al: Affective syndromes, psychotic features, and prognosis, II: mania. Arch Gen Psychiatry 47:658–662, 1990b

Coryell W, Winokur G, Shea T, et al: The long-term stability of depressive subtypes. Am J Psychiatry 151:199–204, 1994

Coryell W, Leon A, Winokur G, et al: Importance of psychotic features to long-term course in major depressive disorder. Am J Psychiatry 153:483–489, 1996

Coryell W, Leon AC, Turvey C, et al: The significance of psychotic features in manic episodes: a report from the NIMH collaborative study. J Affect Disord 67:79–88, 2001

Endicott J, Spitzer RL: A diagnostic interview: the Schedule for Affective Disorders and Schizophrenia. Arch Gen Psychiatry 35:837–844, 1978

Endicott J, Nee J, Coryell W, et al: Schizoaffective, psychotic, and nonpsychotic depression: differential familial association. Compr Psychiatry 27:1–13, 1986

Friedman C, De Mowbray MS, Hamilton V: Imipramine (Tofranil) in depressive states: a controlled trial with inpatients. J Ment Sci 107:948–953, 1961

Glassman AH, Kantor SJ, Shostak M: Depression, delusions, and drug response. Am J Psychiatry 132:716–719, 1975

Hordern A, Holt NF, Burt CG, et al: Amitriptyline in depressive states: phenomenology and prognostic considerations. Br J Psychiatry 109:815–825, 1963

Maser JD, Akiskal HS, Schettler P, et al: Can temperament identify affectively ill patients who engage in lethal or near-lethal suicidal behavior? A 14-year prospective study. Suicide Life Threat Behav 32:10–32, 2002

Roose SP, Glassman AH, Walsh BT, et al: Depression, delusions, and suicide. Am J Psychiatry 140:1159–1162, 1983

Spitzer RL, Endicott J, Robins E: Research Diagnostic Criteria: rationale and reliability. Arch Gen Psychiatry 35:773–782, 1978

CHAPTER 7

Development of Mania or Hypomania in the Course of Unipolar Major Depression

Jess G. Fiedorowicz, M.D., Ph.D.

Jean Endicott, Ph.D.

Hagop S. Akiskal, M.D.

In dealing with unipolar depression, it is necessary to recognize that some patients begin depressed and become bipolar.

Winokur and Tsuang 1996, p. 26

MANIA AND HYPOMANIA serve as defining features of bipolar disorder, a condition characterized by recurrent episodes of mania, hypomania, or depression. These defining syndromes are often not the initial manifestations of illness. Long-term follow-up studies of individuals with unipolar major depression have consistently reported that substantial proportions ultimately experience episodes of mania or hypomania. This conversion suggests that some individuals with the correct diagnosis of unipolar major depression actually have a bipolar disorder, although the defining features of bipolarity have not yet announced themselves. The potential for misclassification with an accurate history presumably carries considerable clinical relevance because the course of illness and treatments for unipolar depression and bipolar disorders differ. Observational studies with intensive follow-up of well-characterized cohorts are required for this relevant clinical issue. We review data from such prospective cohorts, primarily conducted at academic medical centers, and highlight the contributions from the National Institute of Mental Health Collaborative Depression Study (CDS).

Several observational studies have followed up individuals with unipolar major depression diagnoses for the development of mania or hypomania. With the exception of one study reporting 14% conversion after two episodes of depression (Rao and Nammalvar 1977), early (pre-1980) estimates suggested that approximately 5% of individuals presenting with depression would develop mania or hypomania consistent with bipolar disorder (Dunner et al. 1976; Lundquist 1945; Winokur and Morrison 1973). Of interest, early analyses restricted to first-episode depressions found a manic-depressive course in 29%–38% (Kinkelin 1954; Rao and Nammalvar 1977). This higher rate in first episodes was presumed to reflect the common initial presentation of depression in bipolar disorder, and mania was estimated to occur only 20% of the time following three or more initial episodes of depression (Perris 1968). As is detailed later in this chapter, more recent studies have associated recurrent episodes with conversion.

Studies after 1980 generally have reported higher lifetime conversion estimates, likely as a result of closer follow-up and less stringent definitions of mania. Prospective cohort studies that used structured diagnostic interviews of individuals with diagnosed major depressive disorder (MDD) at baseline reported varied rates of diagnostic conversion from unipolar major depression to bipolar disorder of up to 6% a year as detailed in Table 7–1 (Beesdo et al. 2009; Fiedorowicz et al. 2011; Geller et al. 1994; Goldberg et al. 2001; Kovacs et al. 1994; Lehmann et al. 1988; McCauley et al. 1993; Rao et al. 1995; Strober and Carlson 1982; Strober et al. 1993). Although conversion rates are not strictly linear, the percentage of patients changing diagnosis per year of follow-up allows ready comparison of studies. The highest rates of conversion generally have been seen in younger samples (Kovacs 1996), as in the child and adolescent samples highlighted in Table 7–1, in which 2.6%–6.5% progressed to bipolar disorder each year (Geller et al. 1994; Kovacs et al. 1994; McCauley et al. 1993; Rao et al. 1995; Strober and Carlson 1982; Strober et al. 1993). As one might expect, the rate reported by a representative community sample of adolescents and young adults in Germany (Beesdo et al. 2009) appears lower than that observed for clinical samples.

Several samples without a structured baseline assessment reported noteworthy findings. Initial analysis of the Iowa 500 data by Winokur and Morrison (1973) indicated diagnostic conversion at a rate of approximately 1% per year, with 10% of the sample converting later (Winokur and Wesner 1987). In a sample of seriously ill inpatients in Switzerland, the rate of conversion was greatest in the first 4 years after onset of the first episode and thereafter was linear at a change rate of about 1.25% per year (Angst et al. 2005). An outpatient sample studied by Akiskal et al. (1983) showed a 20% conversion rate over 3 years. A mid-study analysis of the CDS after 10 years of follow-up found that approximately 10% of those with diagnosed unipolar depression developed bipolar disorder, a rate of approximately 1% per year (Coryell et al. 1995). Although the summary findings are presented in terms of a conversion rate per year, studies have found that most conversions occur early in the course of depressive illness, with some ongoing risk of conversion to bipolar disorder continuing throughout the illness course.

Several variables are prospectively associated with subsequent mania or hypomania in samples with MDD. Table 7–2 highlights those variables that have been replicated in prospective follow-up of cohorts of subjects with unipolar major depression. For this summary, predictors were counted only once if they appeared in repeat analyses of the same or an overlapping sample. The most consistently replicated predictors include early age at onset (Akiskal et al. 1983; Angst et al. 2005; Beesdo et al. 2009; Fiedorowicz et al. 2011), psychosis (Akiskal et al. 1983; Fiedorowicz et al. 2011; Goldberg et al. 2001; Strober and Carlson 1982; Strober et al. 1993), and a family history of mania (Akiskal et al. 1983; Angst et al. 2005; Fiedorowicz et al. 2011; Strober and Carlson 1982) or a pedigree loaded with mood disorders (Akiskal et al. 1983; Geller et al. 1994; Strober and Carlson 1982). An acute onset of mood syndromes (Akiskal et al. 1995; Strober and Carlson 1982), multiple prior depressive episodes (Angst et al. 2005; Beesdo et al. 2009), hypersomnia or psychomotor retardation (Akiskal et al. 1983; Strober and Carlson 1982), pharmacologically induced hypomania (Akiskal et al. 1983; Strober and Carlson 1982), and subthreshold hypomanic symptoms also have been replicated as predictors of bipolar switching (Fiedorowicz et al. 2011; Zimmermann et al. 2009). Apart from subthreshold hypomanic symptoms, the presence of subtle mixed symptoms has been insufficiently examined. A variety of other variables have been supported by the literature, including, but not limited to, postpartum episodes (Akiskal et al. 1983), chronicity of illness (Coryell et al. 1995), more bodily concerns (Strober and Carlson 1982), decreased concentration (Strober and Carlson 1982), less response to antidepressants (Strober and Carlson 1982), less likely married (Akiskal et al. 1995), and more frequent minor antisocial acts (Akiskal et al. 1995). Personality and temperamental variables also were explored in detail by Akiskal et al. (1995) with the CDS data and are discussed in Chapter 10 ("Personality and Mood Disorders").

TABLE 7–1. Rates of conversion in diagnosis from unipolar depression to bipolar disorder

Study	N	Mean age at intake	Sample acuity	Mean follow-up (years)	Max follow-up (years)	Number of prospective assessments	Bipolar II (%)	Bipolar I (%)	Total conversion (%)	Conversion rate (%/year)
Beesdo et al. 2009	649	14–24[a]	Representative community sample	~ 7[a]	10	3	1.7	2.3	4.0	0.6
Fiedorowicz et al. 2011	550	38	75% inpatient	17.5	31	36	7.5	12.2	19.6	1.1
Geller et al. 1994	79	11	Outpatient	4.9	5	20	19.0	12.7	31.6	6.5
Goldberg et al. 2001	74	23	Inpatient	14.7	15	5	25.7	14.9	40.5	2.8
Kovacs et al. 1994	60	11	Outpatient	6.3	12	Not reported			15.0	2.4
Lehmann et al. 1988	65	42	Inpatient and outpatient	11.3	13	1	0.0	0.0	0.0	0.0
McCauley et al. 1993	65	12	Inpatient and outpatient	3.0	3	4	6.2	1.5	7.7	2.6

TABLE 7–1. Rates of conversion in diagnosis from unipolar depression to bipolar disorder (continued)

Study	N	Mean age at intake	Sample acuity	Mean follow-up (years)	Max follow-up (years)	Number of prospective assessments	Bipolar II (%)	Bipolar I (%)	Total conversion (%)	Conversion rate (%/year)
Rao et al. 1995	26	15	Inpatient <50%	7.0	8	1			19.2	2.7
Strober and Carlson 1982[b]	60	15	Inpatient	3–4	4	6–8	0.0	16.7	16.7	4.2
Strober et al. 1993	58	15	Inpatient	2	2	4			8.6	4.3

Note. This table outlines the results of prospective cohort studies with structured diagnostic interviews at baseline assessing the rate of onset of hypomania or mania in samples with unipolar major depression. Sample size is based on number of individuals with major depression at intake. When a single sample was published several times, the most representative publication was included.
[a]Signifies data provided for entire sample as not specifically reported for subsample with major depressive disorder.
[b]Does not include those who developed mania during index hospitalization.
Source. Adapted and updated from Fiedorowicz et al. 2011

TABLE 7–2. **Replicated predictors of progression from unipolar depression to bipolar disorder**

Variable	Number of studies
Psychosis	5
Early age at onset	4
Family history of bipolar disorder	4
Family history loaded with mood disorders	3
Acute onset of mood syndrome	2
Multiple prior depressive episodes	2
Hypersomnia or psychomotor retardation	2
Pharmacologically induced hypomania	2
Subthreshold hypomanic symptoms	2

Note.   This table highlights variables, replicated in distinct prospective samples, associated with the development of bipolar disorder in individuals diagnosed with unipolar major depression.

Early Collaborative Depression Study Analyses on Progression to Bipolar Disorder

Two mid-study analyses of the CDS described those with unipolar major depression who progressed to bipolar disorder (Akiskal et al. 1995; Coryell et al. 1995). The analysis by Coryell et al. (1995) sought to determine the long-term stability of the diagnostic categories unipolar major depression, bipolar I disorder, and bipolar II disorder. The relevant portions of this analysis selected 381 patients with unipolar major depression at intake who completed 10 years of follow-up. Only 20 (5.2%) of these individuals developed mania, and 19 (5.0%) developed hypomania, and most of these events occurred in the first 5 years of the 10-year follow-up. Overall, baseline diagnosis was strongly predictive of course of illness. Those who progressed to bipolar II disorder tended to be younger at intake and more likely to have had a chronic episode (>2 years in duration) at the time of intake. Those who progressed to bipolar I disorder were more likely to have been psychotic or to have a family history of bipolar I disorder. Coryell et al. (1995) concluded that baseline assessment of polarity was generally stable because 90% remained unipolar.

The second CDS analysis by Akiskal et al. (1995) excluded those with Research Diagnostic Criteria (RDC) schizoaffective disorder because of interest

TABLE 7–3. Clinical correlates of diagnostic conversion from unipolar depression to bipolar disorder in study by Akiskal et al. (1995)

Bipolar I	Bipolar II
More reported feelings of inadequacy and discouragement	Younger age at intake and earlier age at onset
Greater psychic anxiety	Less likely to be married or living with partner
More inability to concentrate	
Greater social withdrawal	Longer duration of index depressive episode
More impaired functioning	
Delusions	Greater likelihood of Research Diagnostic Criteria cyclothymic personality
Hallucinations	More frequent substance use disorder (not alcohol)
	Greater social withdrawal
	More frequent minor antisocial acts
	More likely to have had difficulties with work or school
	More miscellaneous psychopathology

in bipolar II disorder and subsequently observed fewer conversions in diagnosis to bipolar I disorder (3.9%). The Akiskal et al. analysis explored a diverse array of potential predictors of "switching" polarity. Table 7–3 highlights the clinical variables that significantly differentiated subjects who developed bipolar I or II disorder from those who did not change diagnosis.

Akiskal et al. (1995), in their article, explored in depth variables related to temperament and personality. The CDS administered a self-report personality battery that included measures from the Guilford-Zimmerman Temperament Survey (General Activity, Restraint, Ascendance, Sociability, Emotional Stability, Objectivity, and Thoughtfulness), the Interpersonal Dependency Inventory (Emotional Reliance on Another Person, Lack of Social Self-Confidence, Assertion of Autonomy), the Lazare-Klerman-Armor Personality Inventory (Orality, Obsessionality, and Hysterical Pattern), the Maudsley Personality Inventory (Neuroticism and Extraversion), and the Minnesota Multiphasic Personality Inventory (Ego Resiliency and Ego Control–5). Those subjects who developed bipolar II but not bipolar I disorder had several distinguishing features in their personality profile compared with those who did not convert. Those who developed bipolar II disorder had higher scores at intake on measures of Neuroticism, Orality, Emotional Reliance on Another Person, and Lack of Self-Confidence. They scored lower on measures of Ego

Resiliency and Emotional Stability (Akiskal et al. 1995). Akiskal et al. used the aforementioned items to derive composite personality measures that appeared to best discriminate those who developed bipolar II disorder from those with unipolar major depression (and those who developed bipolar I disorder). These variables included mood lability, energy-activity, daydreaming, and insecurity about social encounters (social anxiety). The first three of these had the strongest independent predictive value for converting to bipolar II disorder in analyses that controlled for all other significant predictors. No personality variables were found to characterize subjects who developed bipolar I disorder.

Final Collaborative Depression Study Analysis on Progression to Bipolar Disorder

At the conclusion of the CDS, nearly 1 in 5 (108 of 550; 19.6%) of those with MDD at intake were ultimately reclassified as having a bipolar disorder. In survival analysis, the cumulative probability of developing mania or hypomania was about 1 in 4 (26.3%) (Fiedorowicz et al. 2011). Fiedorowicz et al. identified 550 individuals who had been followed up for at least 1 year and had an intake diagnosis consistent with DSM-IV-TR (American Psychiatric Association 2000) criteria for MDD based on an RDC diagnosis of MDD or schizoaffective disorder, depressed, mainly affective (Fiedorowicz et al. 2011). Of this sample, 7.5% and 12.2% ultimately received rediagnoses of bipolar I disorder and bipolar II disorder, respectively, as highlighted in Figure 7–1. Of those who developed mania at any point, 44% experienced hypomania prior to this mania. Time to develop mania or hypomania/mania is illustrated in the survival curves of Figure 7–2.

At intake, the Schedule for Affective Disorders and Schizophrenia (SADS; Endicott and Spitzer 1978, 1979) screened all participants for five manic symptoms: elevated mood, decreased need for sleep, unusually high energy, increased goal-directed activity, and grandiosity. The Fiedorowicz et al. (2011) analysis focused on assessing the role of subthreshold hypomanic symptoms as predictors of progression to bipolar disorder, while replicating some of the most robust predictors in the established literature: early age at onset, family history of bipolar disorder, and psychosis. Each of these variables appeared to predict progression to bipolar disorder independently. Each subthreshold hypomanic symptom that was present, even when of the lowest intensity rating, was associated with a 24% increased risk (hazard ratio [HR] = 1.24; 95% confidence interval [CI] = 1.09–1.41; $P = 0.001$) of developing bipolar disorder, in-

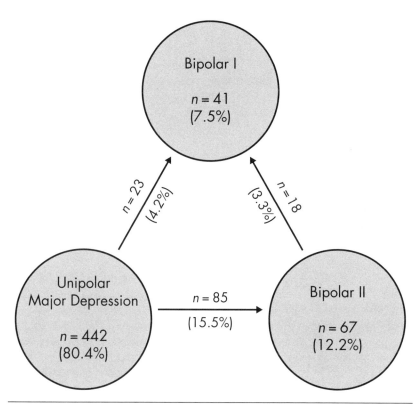

FIGURE 7–1. Progression from unipolar major depression to bipolar disorder in the Collaborative Depression Study (CDS).

Of the 550 individuals with major depressive disorder on intake into the CDS and followed up for at least 1 year, 108 individuals developed mania or hypomania, resulting in a change in diagnosis to bipolar I or bipolar II disorder, respectively. Of those who presented with unipolar major depression, 7.5% developed mania, resulting in a revision of diagnosis to bipolar I disorder. Another 12.2% of the participants developed hypomania without a subsequent mania. The figure shows the progression of changes in diagnosis from this original sample.

dependent of age at onset, family history of bipolar disorder, and psychosis. The presence of at least three subthreshold manic symptoms was identified as an optimal cutoff on a receiver operating characteristic curve but with a sensitivity of only 16%, a specificity of 95%, and a positive predictive value of 42% (Fiedorowicz et al. 2011). These figures suggest that the ability to predict which subjects among those with major depression will progress to bipolar disorder remains limited and underscores the importance of close monitoring of those in treatment.

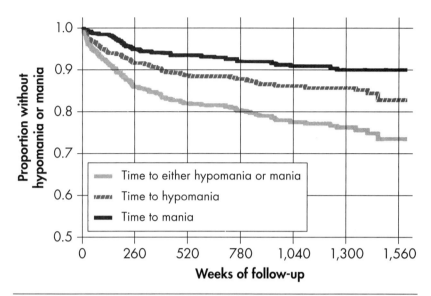

FIGURE 7–2.   Time to progression from unipolar major depression to bipolar disorder in the Collaborative Depression Study.

Over a mean (median) of 17.5 (19.9) and up to 31 years of follow-up, the cumulative probability of progressing to bipolar disorder was 26.3%. Over the first 5 years of follow-up, the rate of change in diagnosis approximated 2.5% per year and thereafter 0.5% per year.

Source.   Reprinted from Fiedorowicz JG, Endicott J, Leon AC, et al.: "Subthreshold Hypomanic Symptoms in Progression From Unipolar Major Depression to Bipolar Disorder." *American Journal of Psychiatry* 168:40–48, 2011. Copyright 2011, American Psychiatric Association. Used with permission.

The predictors of progression to bipolar disorder varied by bipolar subtype in the final analysis (Fiedorowicz et al. 2011). The number of positive manic screens (HR=1.40; 95% CI =1.16–1.68; P=0.0004) and the presence of psychosis at intake (HR=3.54; 95% CI=1.85–6.77; P=0.0001) strongly predicted progression to bipolar I disorder (Fiedorowicz et al. 2011). However, only an earlier age at onset was significantly associated with the development of hypomania in those without any subsequent mania (i.e., those with conversion to bipolar II disorder). The presence of any degree of certain subthreshold hypomanic symptoms (decreased need for sleep, excessive energy, increased goal-directed activity, or grandiosity) was significantly related to development of mania. Decreased need for sleep and excessive energy also were related to the development of hypomania without mania (Fiedorowicz et al. 2011).

Interestingly, the relation between a family history of bipolar disorder and progression from unipolar major depression to bipolar I or bipolar II disorder bred true to the bipolar subtype based on CDS family history data. In the previously referenced sample (Fiedorowicz et al. 2011) of 550 participants with unipolar major depression at intake, 331 had participated in a family study for which 2,467 first-degree biological relatives were interviewed. Another 214 participants had consensus diagnoses for 1,519 first-degree relatives based on the Family History RDC, which used an interview from one or more relatives to establish diagnoses on relatives not interviewed. Family history data were missing for only 5 participants from this sample. A family history of any bipolar disorder was not significantly associated with the development of mania (HR = 1.93; 95% CI = 0.88–4.21; P = 0.10) or hypomania without mania (HR = 1.71; 95% CI = 0.93–3.15; P = 0.08), but a more specific family history of bipolar I or bipolar II disorder was significantly associated with progression to mania (P = 0.02) or hypomania without mania (P = 0.02), respectively. Much earlier analysis of the CDS data had associated diagnosis and family history by bipolar subtype (Coryell et al. 1984). The subsequent analysis confirmed these findings in those who were initially misclassified as having unipolar major depression. In composite, such familiar aggregation by cross-sectional diagnosis and prospective course of illness provides strong empirical support for the validation of the bipolar II subtype.

Follow-Up of Patients With Prospectively Observed New-Onset Mania or Hypomania

The CDS also provided a unique opportunity to perform a follow-up study of prospectively observed new-onset cases of mania or hypomania among those with previously diagnosed unipolar major depression. As previously noted, 108 participants in the CDS began their first episode of mania or hypomania during follow-up. When this initial prospectively observed mania or hypomania was used as the index episode, 60 (56%) went on to have a subsequent manic or hypomanic episode over a mean of 14 additional years of follow-up (Fiedorowicz et al. 2012). Of the 108 who developed mania or hypomania, 21 had a family history of bipolar disorder, and 12 had their first manic or hypomanic episode within 8 weeks of starting an antidepressant or treatment with electroconvulsive therapy. Only 2 of these 12 (17%) had a subsequent manic or hypomanic episode compared with 58 of 96 (60%) of those whose first manic or hypomanic episode did not immediately follow treatment (Fisher exact test, P = 0.005), a significant difference on survival analysis (log-rank test, χ^2_1 = 5.9; P = 0.01). In a multivariate Cox regression model on time to a subsequent mania or hypomania, any family history of bipolar disorder (HR = 2.02; 95%

CI=1.07–3.79; P=0.03) was significantly associated. Treatment-associated hypomania/mania no longer met the threshold for significance (HR=0.24; 95% CI=0.06–1.01; P=0.052). Age at onset also was not related (HR=0.99; 95% CI=0.96–1.02; P=0.37), and duration of the initial hypomanic or manic episode did not predict a repeat episode, whether modeled as 2 weeks or more (HR=0.90; 95% CI=0.46–1.79; P=0.77) or 4 weeks or more (HR=0.91; 95% CI=0.62–1.72; P=0.91). These findings indicate that a family history of bipolar disorder influences course of illness, even after the development of mania or hypomania. Furthermore, duration of a hypomanic or manic episode does not affect the risk of recurrence of similar episodes. The apparent reduced risk of subsequent episodes following treatment-associated hypomania lends some support to those who distinguish treatment-associated hypomania as a distinct disorder on the bipolar spectrum (Akiskal et al. 2003).

Conclusion

With its extended duration and rigorous assessments, the CDS has been uniquely positioned to answer key clinical questions relevant to the progression from unipolar major depression to bipolar disorder. A key strength of the design that facilitated this goal was a thorough baseline assessment that included a structured interview and frequent (every 6 months or 1 year) follow-up assessments. As a result, we now know that approximately one in four adults with unipolar major depression can be expected to develop mania or hypomania and eventually warrant a more appropriate diagnosis of bipolar disorder. The presence of psychosis, an earlier age at onset of affective illness, a family history of the specific bipolar subtype, and the presence of hypomanic symptoms well under the threshold for diagnosis are convincingly established predictors of such progression to bipolar disorder through the CDS.

Prediction models generated from such studies remain insufficient in their ability to reliably identify those patients with a diagnosis of MDD who will progress to bipolar disorder. A valid prediction model would be useful for many purposes. Clinically, it would be important to correctly classify individuals as early as possible for the purpose of treatment selection and counseling the patient and family. For research purposes, an accurate classification of diagnosis is essential for studies of etiology, including genetic studies, and pathophysiology. With approximately one-quarter of those with major depression incorrectly classified, enormous obstacles to many lines of research become evident. Subsequent prospective studies should, in addition to accurate clinical phenotyping and phenomenological assessment, include a genetic profile and data on a variety of salient biomarkers. The resulting data could result in additional predictors and improved identification of individuals likely to progress to bipolar disorder. This research direction may be useful in reclassifying what are likely heterogeneous disorders contained within the rubric of mood disorders, among which useful distinctions beyond polarity or bipolar subtype may be made. The presence of subtle mixed states, either at baseline or during follow-up, has been insufficiently examined in predicting diagnostic conversion. A future challenge in going beyond the current DSM-IV-TR system is to consider the predictive potential of subthreshold mixed states such as "depressive mixed state" (isolated agitated-irritable hypomanic elements as a proxy or predictor for bipolarity) (Akiskal et al. 2005; Benazzi and Akiskal 2001). Prospective longitudinal studies, like the CDS, are essential for addressing these and related nosological questions that are of considerable clinical relevance.

Clinical Implications

- Clinicians should be aware that many of the patients they follow up for what appears to be a unipolar major depression will go on to develop mania or hypomania, the defining syndromes for bipolar disorder. Consequently, close monitoring is critical, particularly for those in the highest risk groups described here. Screening for mania or hypomania should not be limited to the initial evaluation.
- Individuals with a history of psychosis, a family history of bipolar disorder, an earlier age at onset, and subthreshold hypomanic symptoms are at higher risk for developing bipolar disorder. The positive predictive value of these risk factors, however, is limited, and the presence of these risk factors for progression to bipolar disorder does not warrant a change in diagnosis.
- In the Collaborative Depression Study, individuals who developed mania or hypomania following initiation of somatic treatment were less likely to develop a subsequent mania or hypomania. However, these individuals also were older and without psychosis. The nosological relevance of a temporal association with treatment initiation for new-onset mania or hypomania remains unclear.

References

Akiskal HS, Walker P, Puzantian VR, et al: Bipolar outcome in the course of depressive illness: phenomenologic, familial, and pharmacologic predictors. J Affect Disord 5:115–128, 1983

Akiskal HS, Maser JD, Zeller PJ, et al: Switching from 'unipolar' to bipolar II: an 11-year prospective study of clinical and temperamental predictors in 559 patients. Arch Gen Psychiatry 52:114–123, 1995

Akiskal HS, Hantouche EG, Allilaire JF, et al: Validating antidepressant-associated hypomania (bipolar III): a systematic comparison with spontaneous hypomania (bipolar II). J Affect Disord 73:65–74, 2003

Akiskal HS, Benazzi F, Perugi G, et al: Agitated "unipolar" depression re-conceptualized as a depressive mixed state: implications for the antidepressant-suicide controversy. J Affect Disord 85:245–258, 2005

American Psychiatric Association: Diagnostic and Statistical Manual of Mental Disorders, 4th Edition, Text Revision. Washington, DC, American Psychiatric Association, 2000

Angst J, Sellaro R, Stassen HH, et al: Diagnostic conversion from depression to bipolar disorders: results of a long-term prospective study of hospital admissions. J Affect Disord 84:149–157, 2005

Beesdo K, Hofler M, Leibenluft E, et al: Mood episodes and mood disorders: patterns of incidence and conversion in the first three decades of life. Bipolar Disord 11:637–649, 2009

Benazzi F, Akiskal HS: Delineating bipolar II mixed states in the Ravenna-San Diego collaborative study: the relative prevalence and diagnostic significance of hypomanic features during major depressive episodes. J Affect Disord 67:115–122, 2001

Coryell W, Endicott J, Reich T, et al: A family study of bipolar II disorder. Br J Psychiatry 145:49–54, 1984

Coryell W, Endicott J, Maser JD, et al: Long-term stability of polarity distinctions in the affective disorders. Am J Psychiatry 152:385–390, 1995

Dunner DL, Fleiss JL, Fieve RR: The course of development of mania in patients with recurrent depression. Am J Psychiatry 133:905–908, 1976

Endicott J, Spitzer RL: A diagnostic interview: the Schedule for Affective Disorders and Schizophrenia. Arch Gen Psychiatry 35:837–844, 1978

Endicott J, Spitzer RL: Use of the Research Diagnostic Criteria and the Schedule for Affective Disorders and Schizophrenia to study affective disorders. Am J Psychiatry 136:52–56, 1979

Fiedorowicz JG, Endicott J, Leon AC, et al: Subthreshold hypomanic symptoms in progression from unipolar major depression to bipolar disorder. Am J Psychiatry 168:40–48, 2011

Fiedorowicz JG, Endicott J, Solomon DA, et al: Course of illness following prospectively observed mania or hypomania in individuals presenting with unipolar depression. Bipolar Disord 14:664–671, 2012

Geller B, Fox LW, Clark KA: Rate and predictors of prepubertal bipolarity during follow-up of 6- to 12-year-old depressed children. J Am Acad Child Adolesc Psychiatry 33:461–468, 1994

Goldberg JF, Harrow M, Whiteside JE: Risk for bipolar illness in patients initially hospitalized for unipolar depression. Am J Psychiatry 158:1265–1270, 2001

Kinkelin M: [Course and prognosis in manic-depressive psychosis] (in German). Schweiz Arch Neurol Psychiatr 73:100–146, 1954

Kovacs M: Presentation and course of major depressive disorder during childhood and later years of the life span. J Am Acad Child Adolesc Psychiatry 35:705–715, 1996

Kovacs M, Akiskal HS, Gatsonis C, et al: Childhood-onset dysthymic disorder: clinical features and prospective naturalistic outcome. Arch Gen Psychiatry 51:365–374, 1994

Lehmann HE, Fenton FR, Deutsch M, et al: An 11-year follow-up study of 110 depressed patients. Acta Psychiatr Scand 78:57–65, 1988

Lundquist G: Prognosis and course in manic-depressive psychosis. Acta Psychiatr Neurol Suppl 35:1–96, 1945

McCauley E, Myers K, Mitchell J, et al: Depression in young people: initial presentation and clinical course. J Am Acad Child Adolesc Psychiatry 32:714–722, 1993

Perris C: The course of depressive psychoses. Acta Psychiatr Scand 44:238–248, 1968

Rao AV, Nammalvar N: The course and outcome in depressive illness: a follow-up study of 122 cases in Madurai, India. Br J Psychiatry 130:392–396, 1977

Rao U, Ryan ND, Birmaher B, et al: Unipolar depression in adolescents: clinical outcome in adulthood. J Am Acad Child Adolesc Psychiatry 34:566–578, 1995

Strober M, Carlson G: Bipolar illness in adolescents with major depression: clinical, genetic, and psychopharmacologic predictors in a three- to four-year prospective follow-up investigation. Arch Gen Psychiatry 39:549–555, 1982

Strober M, Lampert C, Schmidt S, et al: The course of major depressive disorder in adolescents, I: recovery and risk of manic switching in a follow-up of psychotic and nonpsychotic subtypes. J Am Acad Child Adolesc Psychiatry 32:34–42, 1993

Winokur G, Morrison J: The Iowa 500: follow-up of 225 depressives. Br J Psychiatry 123:543–548, 1973

Winokur G, Tsuang MT: The Natural History of Mania, Depression, and Schizophrenia. Washington, DC, American Psychiatric Press, 1996

Winokur G, Wesner R: From unipolar depression to bipolar illness: 29 who changed. Acta Psychiatr Scand 76:59–63, 1987

Zimmermann P, Bruckl T, Nocon A, et al: Heterogeneity of DSM-IV major depressive disorder as a consequence of subthreshold bipolarity. Arch Gen Psychiatry 66:1341–1352, 2009

Comorbidity of Affective and Substance Use Disorders

Deborah Hasin, Ph.D.
Bari Kilcoyne, B.S.

Studies Prior to the Collaborative Depression Study

Prior to the Collaborative Depression Study (CDS), the comorbidity of depression and substance abuse had been addressed in two main ways. First, the prevalence or levels of depression were examined with a variety of depression measures among substance abusers. Absolute rates or levels of depression varied from study to study, as might be expected given the differences in samples and assessment methods. However, higher levels of depressive symptomatology and rates of depressive disorders were found consistently among substance abuse patients when compared with nonpatient samples (Croughan et al. 1982; Keeler et al. 1979; Pottenger et al. 1978; Rounsaville et al. 1979; Schuckit 1983). Second, studies were conducted to examine substance abuse in samples of psychiatric patients with mixed or unspecified psychiatric disorders (Crowley et al. 1974; Fischer et al.

Dr. Hasin's studies reviewed in this chapter were supported by a NARSAD New Investigators grant (1988–1990) and the New York State Psychiatric Institute. Support for the preparation of this chapter was received from National Institute on Alcohol Abuse and Alcoholism grant K05AA014223 (Hasin) and from the New York State Psychiatric Institute.

1975; Hall et al. 1977; McLellan et al. 1978; Westermeyer and Walzer 1975). These studies generally found high rates of substance abuse. A series of studies also addressed whether unipolar depression could be subtyped into "pure" and "spectrum" disorders by whether a family history of substance abuse was present (Winokur 1979), a topic that has not been pursued more recently.

By the mid-1980s, improvements in diagnostic methods opened up several questions about the relation of substance abuse to well-diagnosed affective disorders. These topics included the prevalence, correlates, and prognostic implications of substance use disorders among patients with affective disorders, considered generally and also by subtype of affective disorder. These questions were addressed in the CDS.

Collaborative Depression Study Advantages for Comorbidity Research

The CDS presented investigators with the first opportunity in the era of phenomenological psychiatry to examine the sociodemographic and clinical correlates of alcohol and drug abuse among patients with different subtypes of affective disorder and to prospectively examine the association between alcoholism and major affective syndromes when diagnosed by specified diagnostic criteria. A number of features of the CDS facilitated this work:

- A large sample of psychiatric patients with affective disorders ($N=955$)
- A multisite study with procedures carefully monitored across sites
- State-of-the-art diagnostic criteria
- State-of-the-art semistructured diagnostic assessment procedures that were carefully developed and pretested for reliability
- Diagnostic assessments administered by clinician interviewers trained in a consistent manner and supervised carefully to maintain individual and cross-site consistency
- Baseline assessments that included dimensional and diagnostic measures
- A longitudinal component that extended over several decades

Features of Research Diagnostic Criteria Substance Use Disorder Diagnoses

The diagnostic nomenclature for substance use disorders used in the CDS merits comment. The substance use disorder diagnoses included "alcoholism" and "drug use disorder." These categories predated DSM-III (American Psychiatric Association 1980) and were diagnosed according to Research Diagnostic Criteria (RDC; Spitzer et al. 1978). The RDC were assessed with the Schedule for Affective Disorders and Schizophrenia (SADS; Endicott and Spitzer 1978), a highly reliable semistructured diagnostic interview designed for clinician interviewers. The SADS-RDC procedure thus diagnosed substance use disorders without differentiating between abuse and dependence. When DSM-III was published, the SADS-RDC procedure for diagnosing alcohol and drug use disorders appeared outdated because it lacked a way to differentiate between abuse and dependence. However, hindsight suggests that the RDC approach, informed by psychometric development methods, was actually prescient because its approach to the diagnosis of substance use disorder is more similar to the substance use disorder criteria proposed for DSM-5 than to any other widely used nomenclature, including the Feighner criteria (Feighner et al. 1972; Kendler et al. 2010), DSM-III-R (American Psychiatric Association 1987), DSM-IV (American Psychiatric Association 1994), and ICD-10 (World Health Organization 1992). Furthermore, variations between the list of RDC for substance use disorder and today's criteria lists may not make a large difference in the diagnosis because latent variable modeling indicates that numerous alcohol-related problems are all observable indicators of a single underlying latent dimension or trait (Compton et al. 2009; Gillespie et al. 2007; Hasin et al. 2012; Krueger et al. 2004; Saha et al. 2006; Shmulewitz et al. 2010; Wu et al. 2009a, 2009b). One difference between SADS-RDC and more recent nomenclatures that warrants mention is that SADS-RDC diagnoses of substance use disorders were only required to have a duration of 1 month or longer. DSM-III-R and DSM-IV required a minimum duration of 1 year during which the minimum number of symptoms occurred. The degree to which this difference led to more frequent diagnoses of substance use disorder in the CDS than would have been found with a longer duration criterion is unknown.

Primary and Other Affective Disorders

Also of relevance to the CDS is the distinction between what is now called primary (or independent) and substance-induced affective disorders. In the CDS and in other studies conducted around the same time, depression was categorized simply as primary or secondary. Although the terms *primary* and *secondary* implied a hierarchy in order of importance, the actual primary and secondary distinction was based simply on which disorder (affective or substance) had the earlier age at onset. More recently, DSM-IV introduced the terms *primary* (independent) and *substance-induced,* the latter for psychiatric disorders occurring in the presence of heavy drinking or drug use. In the DSM-IV system, primary disorders were those that were fully established prior to the onset of substance abuse or that occurred during extended periods of abstinence. Substance-induced disorders, on the contrary, were defined as those that occur during periods of substance use but exceed the expected effects of intoxication or withdrawal or that remit within 1 month after substance use ends.

Prevalence and Correlates of Alcohol and Drug Abuse at Baseline in Collaborative Depression Study Patients

Data from the baseline (intake) interview with CDS patients were used to examine the prevalence and correlates of alcohol and drug abuse (Hasin et al. 1985) (Table 8–1). Current, clinically significant alcohol abuse was found among 23.7% of the sample, and clinically significant drug abuse was found among 9.0%. These rates were much higher than those in the general population; thus, the findings were of particular importance at the time and remain relevant as a benchmark today. The only diagnostic subtype of affective disorder examined in this article, unipolar versus bipolar, was not found to differentiate between patients with or without substance abuse problems. Younger age, male gender, unmarried marital status, and lower socioeconomic status were significantly associated with having alcohol or drug problems at a clinically significant level, whereas a high level of religious involvement, regardless of the denomination, was protective against alcohol or drug problems.

Prospective Course of Alcoholism in Collaborative Depression Study Patients

The course of comorbid alcoholism and depressive disorders has been examined in depth in five articles focused on the subsample of the CDS patients who met RDC for alcoholism at baseline and who participated in the follow-up portion of the CDS (127 of 135 eligible patients, or 94.1%) (Table 8–1). The high retention rate reduced the possibility of attrition bias. RDC alcoholism symptoms among the 127 CDS patients (of whom 112 were inpatients) were compared with those in 123 alcohol rehabilitation inpatients assessed with the same diagnostic procedure (Hasin and Grant 1987; Hasin et al. 1989). The mean number of alcoholism symptoms among the CDS patients was somewhat lower than that among the alcohol rehabilitation inpatients, but the CDS patients represented a group with a wide range in severity of alcoholism (Hasin et al. 1991).

Two-Year Course of Alcoholism

The first prospective CDS of the relation between major affective syndromes and alcoholism examined the 2-year course of alcoholism and a set of time-invariant predictors including characteristics of the affective and alcohol disorders at baseline (Hasin et al. 1989). Survival analyses were used to examine two outcome variables: alcoholism remission (26 or more weeks with no RDC alcoholism symptoms) and subsequent relapse (any recurrence of RDC alcoholism symptoms after at least 26 weeks of remission).

The cumulative probability of remission was 0.67, and among those who experienced remission, the cumulative probability of relapse was 0.29. Of patients whose alcoholism did not remit, 16.7% had died by the 2-year point, half by suicide and the rest, except one, of alcohol-related causes. This high mortality rate underscored the importance of effective treatment of comorbid depression and alcoholism and that the high risk of suicide among such patients remains a current concern (Aharonovich et al. 2002; Niciu et al. 2009).

Some experienced remission from alcoholism soon after the initial evaluation, whereas others experienced remission at later points throughout the 2-year follow-up period. Variables associated with delayed remission included schizoaffective disorder and duration of alcoholism longer than 6 months. In addition, morning drinking and binge drinking were associated with delayed remission. None of the predictors examined were significantly related to the likelihood of relapse.

Five-Year Course of Alcoholism

Two articles were published on the 5-year course of alcoholism. The first article extended the time to 5 years without substantial change in the analytic strategy (Hasin et al. 1991) but added a component examining service use. The second article added an important statistical element to the survival analysis by including the time-varying course of major depression during the 5 years as a predictor of remission and relapse of alcoholism (Hasin et al. 1996a).

At the 5-year point, the cumulative probability of remission lasting at least 6 months among the CDS patients was 0.90, which was higher than at the 2-year point. As expected, given the longer time frame, the cumulative probability of relapse also was higher: 0.50. As was the case at 2-year follow-up, schizoaffective disorder and longer duration of alcoholism at baseline were again significant predictors of poor course of alcoholism (Hasin et al. 1991). Note that the

TABLE 8–1. Studies of substance abuse and affective disorders in the Collaborative Depression Study

Study	Outcomes	Predictors	Time frame	Results	Patient group analyzed
Hasin et al. 1985	Alcohol and drug abuse	Affective disorder; sociodemographic characteristics	Baseline	Higher prevalence of clinically significant alcohol and drug problems was found in the study sample than in nonpatient samples, particularly among those who were male, young, or unmarried or had lower socioeconomic status or lower religious involvement.	Current episode of major affective syndrome ($N=835$)
Hasin et al. 1989	Remission and relapse of alcoholism	Major affective syndromes and alcohol-specific predictors	2-year follow-up	Cumulative probability of remission and relapse was 0.67 and 0.29, respectively. Schizoaffective disorder and alcoholism ≥6 months at baseline predicted longer time to remission. No variable predicted relapse.	Baseline current major affective syndromes and alcoholism ($N=127$)
Hasin et al. 1991	Remission, relapse, and treatment of alcoholism	Major affective syndromes and alcohol-specific predictors	5-year follow-up	Cumulative probability of remission and relapse was 0.90 and 0.50, respectively. Schizoaffective disorder, alcoholism ≥6 months, and greater alcohol dependence severity predicted longer time to remission but not primary and secondary affective distinction. Fewer than 50% of patients were treated for alcoholism, and this was predicted only by social or occupational alcohol problems.	Baseline current major affective syndromes and alcoholism ($N=127$)

TABLE 8–1. Studies of substance abuse and affective disorders in the Collaborative Depression Study (*continued*)

Study	Outcomes	Predictors	Time frame	Results	Patient group analyzed
Mueller et al. 1994	Course of major depressive disorder	Alcoholism	10-year follow-up	Never-alcoholic and past-alcoholic patients had increased likelihood of depression improvement compared with current alcoholic patients.	Major depression and current, past, or no history of alcoholism (*N*=588)
Hasin et al. 1996c	Remission and relapse of major depression	Time-varying status of alcoholism	5-year follow-up	Improvement in alcoholism during follow-up was a strong predictor of better outcome for depression in terms of remission (83.5%) and relapse, regardless of whether the depression was primary or secondary.	Baseline current major affective syndromes and alcoholism (*N*=127)
Hasin et al. 1996a	Remission and relapse of alcoholism	Time-varying status of major depression	5-year follow-up	Improvement in depression during follow-up was a strong predictor of alcoholism remission, but worsening of depression predicted alcoholism relapse. With time-varying depression in the model, schizoaffective disorder was no longer significant, but alcohol dependence severity at baseline remained a significant predictor of poor course.	Baseline current major affective syndromes and alcoholism (*N*=127)

primary and secondary distinction in the affective disorder did not predict course. Although social or occupational problem severity at baseline also did not predict course, severity of a scale of the Edwards Dependence Syndrome symptoms (Edwards and Gross 1976) did predict poor outcome. Once again, no significant time-invariant predictors of relapse were found. Concerning service use, only 46.5% of the patients had any treatment for alcoholism during the 5 years, a low proportion but still much higher than the proportion found in the general population (Hasin et al. 2007). The only significant predictor of alcoholism treatment was severity of social and occupational problems at baseline.

The lack of predictors for alcoholism relapse was a shortcoming of the previous analyses, warranting further investigation by the introduction of time-varying predictors into the analysis (Hasin et al. 1996a). The time-varying status of depression was a significant predictor of remission of alcoholism, a result that was found to be robust in sensitivity analyses that explored whether alternative definitions of the depression time-varying predictor changed the results. Importantly, the time-varying status of depression also was a significant predictor of relapse among patients whose alcoholism had remitted (i.e., the presence of depression predicted the risk of subsequent alcoholism relapse). This result also was robust to different definitions used in sensitivity analyses.

Five-Year Course of Major Depression

The study by Hasin et al. (1996c) addressed the course of major depressive disorder among the 127 CDS patients with current alcoholism and affective disorder at baseline. This study also implemented a time-varying predictor: the time-varying status of RDC alcoholism over the 5 years. In this study, *remission* was defined as at least 8 consecutive weeks without clinically significant symptoms of major depression, and *relapse* was defined as at least 2 consecutive weeks in which clinically significant symptoms of major depression returned. During the 5 years, 83.5% of the patients experienced at least one remission of their depressive disorder.

Survival analysis results indicated that improvement in alcoholism was a strong, significant predictor of the remission of major depression. Furthermore, the time-varying status of alcoholism was a significant predictor of relapse of major depression (i.e., the presence of alcoholism increased the likelihood of depression relapse). Neither the primary and secondary distinction in the depressive disorder nor the covarying status of drug disorder was a significant predictor of the course of the depressive disorder.

Ten-Year Course of Major Depression

One study examined whether alcoholism influenced the course of major depression over 10 years of follow-up (Mueller et al. 1994) (Table 8–1). This study used a different design, including groups of patients defined at baseline with no prior alcoholism, remitted alcoholism, or current alcoholism. Furthermore, patients with a history of bipolar or schizoaffective disorder at baseline were excluded to focus more closely on unipolar depression. In this study, the investigators wanted to examine all transitions into and out of depression rather than limit the analyses to the initial transitions into remission and subsequent relapse, as is done in survival analysis. The study predated the current widespread use of general linear mixed effects models, now the standard method for investigating such multiple transitions over time and their predictors that takes into account within-subject correlations over time. The investigators used a novel statistical method that they termed *intensity analysis*. Study findings indicated that past or inactive alcoholism did not confer a risk for poor course of depression (transitions from well to ill with regard to depression, or failure to transition from ill to well). However, current alcoholism was a strong, significant predictor of transitions from well to ill and failure to transition from ill to well.

Effect of Collaborative Depression Study Results on Subsequent Research on Affective and Substance Disorders

CDS studies on the comorbidity of affective and substance use disorders clearly indicated that among patients in treatment for clinically severe affective syndromes, alcohol and drug problems were common and that the course of the affective and substance disorders was intertwined to a substantial extent. Since publication of the last of this set of papers 16 years ago, the work has been cited in subsequent peer-reviewed papers more than 200 times.

Perhaps the most direct influence of this work on comorbidity research was a National Institute on Drug Abuse–funded prospective study of the course of comorbid affective and substance use disorders, termed the *Clinfol study* (Hasin et al. 2002), that derived many of its elements directly from the CDS. Among its subsamples, this study included 250 psychiatric inpatients with affective and/ or anxiety disorders and comorbid heavy drinking or drug use and carefully differentiated between primary and substance-induced major depressive episodes according to DSM-IV definitions. The Clinfol study used improved diagnostic measures (Hasin et al. 1996b, 2006) that grew out of the experience of the CDS and that provided highly reliable diagnoses of psychiatric disorders among patients who were heavy drinkers or drug users. By design, many patients in the Clinfol study had cocaine or heroin dependence as well as alcohol dependence.

These patients were selected in part because of the degree of interest in how the courses of affective disorders and these additional substances were related and in part because of the importance of eliminating "substance substitution" as a potential artifactual explanation of seeming remissions in the course of a single substance use (Hasin et al. 2002). The Clinfol study showed again that time-varying predictors are important components of analysis of the course of a given condition. Results indicated that the course of major depression and substance use disorders was highly intertwined (Hasin et al. 2002; Nunes et al. 2006; Samet et al. 2013). Initial results showed that the time-varying course of major depression was an important predictor of the longitudinal course of a combined substance outcome (i.e., alcohol, cocaine, and/or heroin dependence) (Hasin et al. 2002). Similar results were obtained when alcohol, cocaine, and heroin dependence were considered as separate outcomes (Samet et al. 2013). Interestingly, in the Clinfol study, many substance-induced major depressive disorder diagnoses at baseline were recategorized to independent major depressive disorder over a 12-month follow-up period (Nunes et al. 2006).

The CDS study of substance and affective comorbidity did not address the issue of cannabis, almost certainly because the clinical relevance of cannabis use was seen differently at the inception of the CDS than it is today. The use of cannabis is increasing in the general population (Monitoring the Future 2011), the potency of the cannabis available today in terms of delta-9-tetrahydrocannabinol (its active ingredient) is much stronger than the cannabis that was available at the start of the CDS (ElSohly et al. 2000; Mehmedic et al. 2010), and a cannabis withdrawal syndrome has been documented in laboratory, clinical, and epidemiological studies (Budney et al. 2004; Hasin et al. 2008). At the same time, social norms regarding the acceptability of cannabis use (Keyes et al. 2011) are becoming more positive. Sixteen states now have laws allowing the use of marijuana for medical purposes, and these states have higher rates of marijuana use, abuse, and dependence than do other states (Cerda et al. 2012; Wall et al. 2011). Therefore, this is an issue of comorbidity that has become much more prominent since patients entered the CDS in 1978–1981. Patients with affective disorders may see marijuana as a positive alternative to pharmacological intervention for mood, appetite, or sleep disturbance. A recent case report (Nussbaum et al. 2011) suggested the potential risks for such marijuana use when not adequately monitored. The Clinfol study indicated that among patients hospitalized with nonpsychotic disorders (largely affective) in a dual-diagnosis psychiatric unit, postdischarge cannabis use predicted poor course of alcohol, cocaine, and heroin dependence (Aharonovich et al. 2005). In a different study in a substance abuse research clinic, cannabis dependence was highly associated with independent (primary) depression (Dakwar et al. 2011). Thus, future directions in the comorbidity of affective and substance use disorders should include the issue of cannabis use, which warrants clinical attention and more extensive focus in research.

Clinical Implications

- Although the baseline data indicated lower mean severity of alcoholism symptoms among Collaborative Depression Study patients than among alcohol rehabilitation patients, more than a quarter of the CDS patients had comorbid alcohol and/or drug problems. This high prevalence underscores the need to screen carefully for substance use problems when first evaluating patients entering treatment for affective disorders, even among patients who might not initially seem to be "the type" to have substance use problems.

- Perhaps one of the most important findings from the series of CDS studies described here was the degree to which the time-varying course of depression affected the status of alcoholism and the time-varying status of alcoholism-affected depression. The findings suggest that clinicians treating major depression should assess for and treat comorbid alcoholism in their patients to achieve a good outcome of the depressive disorder. Achieving a good outcome of the alcoholism is important as well.

- The CDS results showed that a high proportion of patients with current alcoholism at baseline experienced remission of alcoholism. Clinicians should therefore feel a reasonable degree of optimism about the chances for a sustained remission of alcoholism among patients with affective disorders. Furthermore, the chances for such remissions can be improved through the use of evidence-based treatments for alcoholism, including pharmacological treatments such as naltrexone (Petrakis et al. 2007) and behavioral treatments such as cognitive-behavioral treatment focused on relapse prevention (Carroll et al. 1994). Both types of treatment have been shown to be safe and effective among individuals with major depression and thus should be considered when planning the treatment regimen.

- The CDS provided a unique opportunity to better understand the course of affective and substance use disorders over time, providing an important stimulus to research and information to guide clinical treatment.

References

Aharonovich E, Liu X, Nunes E, et al: Suicide attempts in substance abusers: effects of major depression in relation to substance use disorders. Am J Psychiatry 159:1600–1602, 2002

Aharonovich E, Liu X, Samet S, et al: Postdischarge cannabis use and its relationship to cocaine, alcohol, and heroin use: a prospective study. Am J Psychiatry 162:1507–1514, 2005

American Psychiatric Association: Diagnostic and Statistical Manual of Mental Disorders, 3rd Edition. Washington, DC, American Psychiatric Association, 1980

American Psychiatric Association: Diagnostic and Statistical Manual of Mental Disorders, 3rd Edition, Revised. Washington, DC, American Psychiatric Association, 1987

American Psychiatric Association: Diagnostic and Statistical Manual of Mental Disorders, 4th Edition. Washington, DC, American Psychiatric Association, 1994

Budney AJ, Hughes JR, Moore BA, et al: Review of the validity and significance of cannabis withdrawal syndrome. Am J Psychiatry 161:1967–1977, 2004

Carroll KM, Rounsaville BJ, Gordon LT, et al: Psychotherapy and pharmacotherapy for ambulatory cocaine abusers. Arch Gen Psychiatry 51:177–187, 1994

Cerda M, Wall M, Keyes KM, et al: Medical marijuana laws in 50 states: investigating the relationship between state legalization of medical marijuana and marijuana use, abuse and dependence. Drug Alcohol Depend 120:22–27, 2012

Compton WM, Saha TD, Conway KP, et al: The role of cannabis use within a dimensional approach to cannabis use disorders. Drug Alcohol Depend 100:221–227, 2009

Croughan JL, Miller JP, Wagelin D, et al: Psychiatric illness in male and female narcotic addicts. J Clin Psychiatry 43:225–228, 1982

Crowley TJ, Chesluk D, Dilts S, et al: Drug and alcohol abuse among psychiatric admissions: a multidrug clinical-toxicologic study. Arch Gen Psychiatry 30:13–20, 1974

Dakwar E, Nunes EV, Bisaga A, et al: A comparison of independent depression and substance-induced depression in cannabis-, cocaine-, and opioid-dependent treatment seekers. Am J Addict 20:441–446, 2011

Edwards G, Gross MM: Alcohol dependence: provisional description of a clinical syndrome. BMJ 1:1058–1061, 1976

ElSohly MA, Ross SA, Mehmedic Z, et al: Potency trends of delta9-THC and other cannabinoids in confiscated marijuana from 1980–1997. J Forensic Sci 45:24–30, 2000

Endicott J, Spitzer RL: A diagnostic interview: the Schedule for Affective Disorders and Schizophrenia. Arch Gen Psychiatry 35:837–844, 1978

Feighner JP, Robins E, Guze SB, et al: Diagnostic criteria for use in psychiatric research. Arch Gen Psychiatry 26:57–63, 1972

Fischer DE, Halikas JA, Baker JW, et al: Frequency and patterns of drug abuse in psychiatric patients. Dis Nerv Syst 36:550–553, 1975

Gillespie NA, Neale MC, Prescott CA, et al: Factor and item-response analysis DSM-IV criteria for abuse of and dependence on cannabis, cocaine, hallucinogens, sedatives, stimulants and opioids. Addiction 102:920–930, 2007

Hall RC, Popkin MK, Devaul R, et al: The effect of unrecognized drug abuse on diagnosis and therapeutic outcome. Am J Drug Alcohol Abuse 4:455–465, 1977

Hasin DS, Grant BF: Psychiatric diagnosis of patients with substance abuse problems: a comparison of two procedures, the DIS and the SADS-L: alcoholism, drug abuse/dependence, anxiety disorders and antisocial personality disorder. J Psychiatr Res 21:7–22, 1987

Hasin D, Endicott J, Lewis C: Alcohol and drug abuse in patients with affective syndromes. Compr Psychiatry 26:283–295, 1985

Hasin DS, Endicott J, Keller MB: RDC alcoholism in patients with major affective syndromes: two-year course. Am J Psychiatry 146:318–323, 1989

Hasin DS, Endicott J, Keller MB: Alcohol problems in psychiatric patients: 5-year course. Compr Psychiatry 32:303–316, 1991

Hasin D, Tsai WY, Endicott J, et al: The effects of major depression on alcoholism: five-year course. Am J Addict 5:144–155, 1996a

Hasin DS, Trautman KD, Miele GM, et al: Psychiatric Research Interview for Substance and Mental Disorders (PRISM): reliability for substance abusers. Am J Psychiatry 153:1195–1201, 1996b

Hasin DS, Tsai WY, Endicott J, et al: Five-year course of major depression: effects of comorbid alcoholism. J Affect Disord 41:63–70, 1996c

Hasin D, Liu X, Nunes E, et al: Effects of major depression on remission and relapse of substance dependence. Arch Gen Psychiatry 59:375–380, 2002

Hasin D, Samet S, Nunes E, et al: Diagnosis of comorbid psychiatric disorders in substance users assessed with the Psychiatric Research Interview for Substance and Mental Disorders for DSM-IV. Am J Psychiatry 163:689–696, 2006

Hasin DS, Stinson FS, Ogburn E, et al: Prevalence, correlates, disability, and comorbidity of DSM-IV alcohol abuse and dependence in the United States: results from the National Epidemiologic Survey on Alcohol and Related Conditions. Arch Gen Psychiatry 64:830–842, 2007

Hasin DS, Keyes KM, Alderson D, et al: Cannabis withdrawal in the United States: results from NESARC. J Clin Psychiatry 69:1354–1363, 2008

Hasin DS, Fenton MC, Beseler C, et al: Analyses related to the development of DSM-5 criteria for substance use related disorders, 2: proposed DSM-5 criteria for alcohol, cannabis, cocaine and heroin disorders in 663 substance abuse patients. Drug Alcohol Depend 122:28–37, 2012

Keeler MH, Taylor CI, Miller WC: Are all recently detoxified alcoholics depressed? Am J Psychiatry 136:586–588, 1979

Kendler KS, Munoz RA, Murphy G: The development of the Feighner criteria: a historical perspective. Am J Psychiatry 167:134–142, 2010

Keyes KM, Schulenberg JE, O'Malley PM, et al: The social norms of birth cohorts and adolescent marijuana use in the United States, 1976–2007. Addiction 106:1790–1800, 2011

Krueger RF, Nichol PE, Hicks BM, et al: Using latent trait modeling to conceptualize an alcohol problems continuum. Psychol Assess 16:107–119, 2004

McLellan AT, Druley KA, Carson JE: Evaluation of substance abuse problems in a psychiatric hospital. J Clin Psychiatry 39:425–430, 1978

Mehmedic Z, Chandra S, Slade D, et al: Potency trends of Delta9-THC and other cannabinoids in confiscated cannabis preparations from 1993 to 2008. J Forensic Sci 55:1209–1217, 2010

Monitoring the Future: Marijuana: Trends in Annual Use, Risk, Disapproval, and Availability: Grades 8, 10, and 12. 2011. Available at: http://monitoringthefuture.org/data/11data/fig11_1.pdf. Accessed March 2, 2012.

Mueller TI, Lavori PW, Keller MB, et al: Prognostic effect of the variable course of alcoholism on the 10-year course of depression. Am J Psychiatry 151:701–706, 1994

Niciu MJ, Chan G, Gelernter J, et al: Subtypes of major depression in substance dependence. Addiction 104:1700–1709, 2009

Nunes EV, Liu X, Samet S, et al: Independent versus substance-induced major depressive disorder in substance-dependent patients: observational study of course during follow-up. J Clin Psychiatry 67:1561–1567, 2006

Nussbaum A, Thurstone C, Binswanger I: Medical marijuana use and suicide attempt in a patient with major depressive disorder. Am J Psychiatry 168:778–781, 2011

Petrakis I, Ralevski E, Nich C, et al: Naltrexone and disulfiram in patients with alcohol dependence and current depression. J Clin Psychopharmacol 27:160–165, 2007

Pottenger M, McKernon J, Patrie LE, et al: The frequency and persistence of depressive symptoms in the alcohol abuser. J Nerv Ment Dis 166:562–570, 1978

Rounsaville BJ, Weissman MM, Rosenberger PH, et al: Detecting depressive disorders in drug abusers: a comparison of screening instruments. J Affect Disord 1:255–267, 1979

Saha TD, Chou SP, Grant BF: Toward an alcohol use disorder continuum using item response theory: results from the National Epidemiologic Survey on Alcohol and Related Conditions. Psychol Med 36:931–941, 2006

Samet S, Fenton MC, Nunes E, et al: Effects of independent and substance-induced major depressive disorder on remission and relapse of alcohol and heroin dependence. Addiction 108(1):115–123, 2013

Schuckit MA: Alcoholic men with no alcoholic first-degree relatives. Am J Psychiatry 140:439–443, 1983

Shmulewitz D, Keyes K, Beseler C, et al: The dimensionality of alcohol use disorders: results from Israel. Drug Alcohol Depend 111:146–154, 2010

Spitzer RL, Endicott J, Robins E: Research Diagnostic Criteria: rationale and reliability. Arch Gen Psychiatry 35:773–782, 1978

Wall MM, Poh E, Cerda M, et al: Adolescent marijuana use from 2002 to 2008: higher in states with medical marijuana laws, cause still unclear. Ann Epidemiol 21:714–716, 2011

Westermeyer J, Walzer V: Socioathy and drug use in a young psychiatric population. Dis Nerv Syst 36:673–677, 1975

Winokur G: Unipolar depression: is it divisible into autonomous subtypes? Arch Gen Psychiatry 36:47–52, 1979

World Health Organization: International Statistical Classification of Diseases and Related Health Problems, 10th Revision (ICD-10). Geneva, Switzerland, World Health Organization, 1992

Wu LT, Pan JJ, Blazer DG, et al: The construct and measurement equivalence of cocaine and opioid dependences: a National Drug Abuse Treatment Clinical Trials Network (CTN) study. Drug Alcohol Depend 103:114–123, 2009a

Wu LT, Pan JJ, Blazer DG, et al: An item response theory modeling of alcohol and marijuana dependences: a National Drug Abuse Treatment Clinical Trials Network study. J Stud Alcohol Drugs 70:414–425, 2009b

CHAPTER 9

Treatment Effectiveness and Safety in the Longitudinal Course of Mood Disorders

Jess G. Fiedorowicz, M.D., Ph.D.

CLINICAL TRIALS are widely considered the gold standard in determining treatment effectiveness but are not without limitations and are unable to address questions that preclude randomization. In some circumstances, randomization would not be ethical, and in others, uncommon outcomes would require prohibitively large sample sizes or unfeasible durations of follow-up. The inclusion and exclusion criteria imposed by trials also limit generalizability. Observational studies supplement the findings of randomized controlled trials by examining treatment effectiveness in broader samples (Leon and Hedeker 2005).

The Collaborative Depression Study (CDS) observed, but did not direct, treatment and thus avoided ethical concerns related to randomization with-

This chapter is dedicated to Andrew C. Leon, Ph.D., who developed the methods behind and led several of the studies highlighted in this chapter and whose untimely death preceded its writing. The author is also indebted to Chunshan (Charles) Li, Research Biostatistician at Weill Medical College at Cornell University, who worked closely with Dr. Leon.

out clinical equipoise. The CDS sample also was large, and participants were followed up for as long as 31 years. Few clinical trials could match the size of the CDS cohort, and certainly none could match the duration of follow-up because the cost would be prohibitive, and the treatments to which individuals were randomly assigned would have long been discontinued for the vast majority of participants. The CDS, although selecting for those with more severe forms of affective illness and involving a predominantly inpatient sample at intake, provided a broadly generalizable sample, including individuals at high risk for suicide, those with substance use, and those being treated in a variety of treatment settings. Without randomization, however, observational studies such as the CDS must use rigorous methods to mitigate the effects of confounding because treatment selection is not randomly assigned, and a variety of factors may influence the decisions involved in seeking, being prescribed, and ultimately taking somatic therapies. The availability of such methods to address this confounding evolved over the more than 30-year course of the CDS, and state-of-the art methods were applied to address the issue of treatment effectiveness in observational studies and disentangle the effects from the determinants of treatment.

Maintenance Treatment With Antidepressants

CDS investigators used long-term follow-up to address questions about maintenance therapy with antidepressants in the early 1990s, at which time data to guide practice were very sparse (Dawson et al. 1998; Lavori et al. 1994). After achieving a remission from depression with an antidepressant medication, persons with major depressive disorder and their providers are faced with a difficult decision. Should treatment be continued, and if so, for how long and at what dose? A prior trial by Frank et al. (1990) suggested benefit to continuing antidepressants up to 17 weeks after remission, although there was some debate as to whether this was a result of protection from continued imipramine or relapse triggered by its withdrawal. A follow-up of 20 participants from this original maintenance trial between years 3 and 5 suggested benefit of full-dose imipramine, although comparisons with lower doses were lacking (Kupfer et al. 1992). General practice, as observed in the CDS, suggested that clinicians slowly tapered antidepressants following remission. The proportion receiving the highest doses of antidepressants declined from 30% the first week of remission to 19% at 6 months, 13% at 1 year, and 9% at 2 years (Lavori et al. 1994). The proportion receiving no antidepressants rose from 37% in the first week of remission to 53% at 6 months, 67% at 1 year, and 74% at 2 years (Lavori et al. 1994). Clinical practice appeared to rest on the assumption that lower doses were adequate for maintenance, which was continued for varied durations.

At the 5-year follow-up of the CDS, Lavori et al. (1994) selected a sample of 339 individuals with unipolar major depression who had clearly recovered from their index episode. The intensity of antidepressant treatment was assessed with the Unipolar Composite Antidepressant (UCAD) treatment score, including four combinations of somatic therapies (Keller et al. 1992). Examples of thresholds for this rating are shown in Table 9–1, adapted from Leon et al. (2003). The analysis addressed the effect of confounding factors on treatment through adjustment by a propensity score, an estimate of the likelihood of receiving a treatment. This propensity score is derived in logistic regression by using available variables and addresses the fact that specific individuals may be more or less likely to receive a treatment. The factors that determine who is prescribed a treatment, such as type or severity of illness, may influence outcomes. Use of a propensity score to control for confounding factors related to medication selection was relatively new in the broader medical literature and was previously unknown in the psychiatric literature (Lavori et al. 1994). The risk of recurrence was modeled to address the time-varying nature of treatment. These methods also facilitated the investigation of a variety of predictors of recurrence, many of which are relevant to the aforementioned clinical questions that are regularly faced by care providers. In developing the propensity score, Lavori et al. found that those who stopped antidepressants during remission indeed differed on several important variables compared with those who continued treatment in that they had experienced fewer prior episodes, had shorter index episodes, were younger at intake, and were more likely to have received treatment as an inpatient. As might be expected given that those at higher risk may be more likely to maintain treatments, adjusting for the propensity score augmented the apparent beneficial effect of antidepressants on preventing recurrence. The study found that continuing antidepressants in the first 6 months following remission reduced risks of recurrence, and further continuation (beyond 6 months) appeared to provide no additional benefit.

Dawson et al. (1998) expanded the findings of Lavori et al. to address the question of antidepressant dosing during maintenance treatment. One prior trial had used two doses of phenelzine and had found no significant differences between 60 and 45 mg/day, although results suggested some advantage of the former (Robinson et al. 1991). In the Dawson et al. analysis, the level of antidepressant was assessed with the UCAD, as in the Lavori et al. study (Keller et al. 1992), and most CDS participants had a slow (weeks to months) decrease in the intensity of antidepressant pharmacology following remission. Those who maintained the same dose of medication used to achieve remission, based on the dose at the end of the index episode, were compared with those who continued antidepressants at lower doses than those used to

TABLE 9–1. Unipolar Composite Antidepressant ratings for selected antidepressants

Somatic treatment	1	2	3	4
Bupropion	1–149	150–299	300–449	≥450
Citalopram	1–19	20–39	40–59	≥60
Fluoxetine	1–10	11–20	21–30	>30
Imipramine	1–99	100–199	200–299	≥300
Mirtazapine	1–14	15–29	30–44	≥45
Paroxetine	1–19	20–39	40–59	≥60
Phenelzine	1–29	30–59	60–74	≥75
Sertraline	1–49	50–100	101–199	≥200
Tranylcypromine	1–19	20–49	50–64	≥65
Trazodone	1–199	200–399	400–599	≥600
Venlafaxine	1–108	109–241	242–374	≥375

Source.   Adapted from Leon et al. 2003.

achieve remission. Individuals who remained on the same dose were at lower risk for recurrence than were those maintained at lower doses. This benefit appeared to extend beyond 6 months to approximately 8 months and beyond 1 year for those with five or more previous episodes (Dawson et al. 1998). Given the limited number of individuals maintaining antidepressant therapy at the dose used to achieve remission, statistical power was limited beyond these durations. The results yielded essential, clinically applicable guidance about the importance of keeping all patients on the level of somatotherapy used to treat the acute episode for the initial 8 months after symptoms have abated (Dawson et al. 1998).

The findings of Lavori et al. and Dawson et al. helped to inform subsequent controlled trials. Longer maintenance trials followed, but given issues related to cost and feasibility, few extended beyond 12 months. A meta-analysis of pooled data from 31 such trials has found that antidepressants are protective and reduce the relative risk of relapse by approximately 70% (Geddes et al. 2003). Although the relative risk reduction remains similar, the absolute risk of relapse in the first 12 months is twice that in subsequent months (Geddes et al. 2003). This may explain why it is difficult to show benefit at greater durations. Not only is statistical power decreased because of a declining portion of the sample receiving full-dose treatment, but also the absolute risk reduction is smaller.

Nonetheless, observational data from the CDS certainly provided evidence that a longer duration of maintenance than was routinely being provided in practice was beneficial, particularly at the full dose required for remission.

Solomon et al. (2005) used CDS data for participants followed up to 20 years and went on to study the phenomenon of recurrence despite maintenance treatment with antidepressant medications. For this analysis, the sample was restricted to 103 individuals who had recovered from their intake episode, had at least one subsequent recurrence, recovered from this prospectively observed episode, and received adequate antidepressant maintenance pharmacotherapy, on the basis of a UCAD score of 3 or greater on the 4-point scale. From these 103 participants, a total of 171 maintenance treatment intervals were identified. These intervals lasted a median of 20 weeks, and recurrence was identified in 42 (25%) of these episodes at a median of 31 weeks. Mixed models were used to allow multiple observations per subjects with varied numbers of observations between subjects. When contrasting maintenance treatment intervals with and without relapse, Solomon et al. found no relation to duration of the prior episode, number of lifetime episodes, lifetime history of alcohol dependence, co-occurring anxiety disorders, or the presence of psychosis. However, individuals with the melancholic subtype of major depression (Research Diagnostic Criteria endogenous major depressive disorder) were approximately 2.5 times as likely to experience a recurrence during maintenance pharmacotherapy ($P < 0.02$), and severity of the prior episode was marginally associated with risk of recurrence ($P < 0.07$) (Solomon et al. 2005).

Maintenance Treatment With Lithium

Akin to the concern about recurrence during maintenance treatment of unipolar major depression with antidepressant medications was interest in recurrence during maintenance treatment of bipolar disorder with lithium. One large, long-term (2-year) randomized controlled trial of lithium versus imipramine for the treatment of bipolar disorder showed benefit of lithium over imipramine (Prien et al. 1984). Another trial that followed up participants for up to 1.5 years found that standard-dose lithium (0.8–1.0 mmol/L) was superior to low-dose lithium (0.4–0.6 mmol/L), which carried a risk of relapse that was 2.6 times higher than that with the standard dose (Gelenberg et al. 1989). Studies of lithium discontinuation without abrupt cessation to support sustained prophylactic benefit were lacking. In a larger CDS sample, Coryell et al. (1997) investigated the long-term benefit of lithium therapy. For the 139 individuals taking lithium compared with the 42 who were not, a survival benefit favored lithium in preventing recurrence in the first 8 months. No such benefit could be seen in the 86 individuals taking lithium compared with the 22 not taking lithium in the period following 8 months. Treatment assignment was, of course, not random, and those who received lithium were more likely to have been inpatients at intake, to have presented with mania, to have a family history of mania, and to have been given an antipsychotic following recovery. Given the apparent greater severity for the lithium-treated group, Coryell et al. (1997) thus concluded that treatment differences may have limited the ability to detect prophylactic benefits of lithium, and they invited randomized controlled trials of gradual lithium discontinuation in those with at least 8 months of sustained euthymia.

Around the same time, another debate was brewing related to case reports suggesting that the discontinuation of lithium led to a subsequent resistance to its therapeutic effects. One observational study attempted to test this hypothesis and showed no evidence of greater morbidity across two separate treatment periods with lithium (Tondo et al. 1997). Coryell et al. (1998) identified 28 individuals from the CDS sample with separate lithium treatment intervals. Between these intervals, participants had been without lithium for a mean of almost 1 year (50 weeks). Comparisons using survival analysis on both time to recovery for the index and first prospectively observed episode during lithium treatment and time to recurrence during lithium prophylaxis were nearly identical between these groups (Coryell et al. 1998). These results did not support the apparent false alarm provoked by case series data of the potential deleterious effects of lithium discontinuation on subsequent therapeutic benefit.

Statistical Methods for Comparison of Nonequivalent Groups Over Long-Term Follow-Up

As the duration of the CDS grew to encompass up to 31 years of prospective follow-up, methods had to be developed to maximally use these long-term data. Across decades of follow-up, participants often endured multiple mood episodes and may have had several treatment trials. Looking at index or first prospectively observed episodes now merely scratched the surface of the data. It also had become more complicated to address confounding through covariate adjustment. Baseline variables may no longer be relevant, and the assumption of proportional hazards grew more tenuous over decades of follow-up. Statistical methods had to deal with not only the variables influencing the propensity to receive treatment but also the fact that participants had numerous treatment intervals and that these treatment intervals were not independent observations. Maximal use of these longitudinal data required inclusion of multiple treatment intervals. Yet most traditional statistical methods assume that observations are independent. The analysis of several presumably correlated treatment intervals for individual participants would violate the assumption of independent observations.

CDS collaborator and biostatistician Andrew C. Leon developed statistical methods that allowed CDS data to answer important questions about treatment effectiveness and safety (Leon and Hedeker 2005; Leon et al. 2001). These methods required a change in the fundamental unit by which the data were viewed. Instead of individual participants representing the unit of analysis or the "rows" of observations to be analyzed, alternative units of analysis could be used, such as mood episodes or treatment intervals. For example, instead of assessing the relation between antidepressants and suicide in 757 participants with mood disorders, Leon et al. (2011) examined this relation in 6,716 treatment intervals in a seminal study that is detailed later in this chapter. This methodological approach poses distinct advantages. Mood disorders tend to be episodic, and an afflicted individual's clinical condition is often in dynamic flux. Instead of controlling for individual covariates that may be broadly relevant, the use of treatment intervals as the unit of analysis allows one to build variables into the propensity score that determines not only the likelihood of receiving treatment but also the likelihood of receiving treatment at that particular point in time. The CDS data provided a tremendous opportunity to apply these methods. Although several large pharmacoepidemiological studies have used propensity scores to investigate the effects of treatment, variables that capture varying severity of illness are often lacking. The CDS data provided weekly ratings describing both the severity and the trajectory of mood symptoms, information that is highly relevant clinically to treatment selection and that has been confirmed as such empirically in the CDS and other data (Leon et al. 2011, 2012; Prabhakar et al. 2011).

Once data were reformatted to a unit of analysis other than the individual participant, these statistical methods invoked a two-stage process. The first stage involved building a propensity score, akin to the aforementioned pioneering work of Lavori et al. (1994) on applying a propensity score to study effectiveness of antidepressant maintenance therapies. Treatment intervals then could be matched for comparison, such that episodes with a similar likelihood of receiving treatment were compared. The second stage invoked a mixed-effects, grouped-time survival analysis. This method allows for inclusion of multiple episodes from the same participant. To facilitate this, time must be grouped based on clinical criteria and treated as an ordinal variable instead of a continuous measure. The overall method addresses confounding by indication, wherein the indication for treatment (e.g., severe or worsening depression) affects risk of the outcome (e.g., suicide) through use of the propensity score based on current clinical and sociodemographic data. The method also maximizes the use of long-term data by providing a mechanism for dealing with correlated observations. Several analyses led by Dr. Leon used related methods to address the effectiveness and safety of pharmacotherapies for mood disorders.

Antidepressant Safety

Many clinical trials have confirmed the efficacy of antidepressant pharmacotherapy, but questions remained regarding whether these results were broadly generalizable. The CDS cohort included individual adults of all ages, including the elderly, as well as those with severe forms of illness (suicidal ideation or psychotic symptoms) and co-occurring medical and psychiatric conditions. Participants also took a variety of antidepressants and dosages. From these data, Leon et al. (2003) developed a propensity score for antidepressant treatment intensity based on the UCAD. Sociodemographic variables were not relevant to the propensity to receive intensive treatment, whereas clinical variables such as number of prior affective episodes, severity of symptoms, trajectory of symptoms, and treatment intensity during the prior episode and prior well interval were. Propensity scores were calculated for each treatment interval, which served as the unit of analysis. The rich CDS data on severity and course of illness provided a rare opportunity to develop a propensity score using such clinical data (Prabhakar et al. 2011). After development of this propensity score, mixed-effect, grouped-time survival analyses were conducted, stratified by propensity score quintile to match those episodes at similar likelihood of receiving treatment (Leon et al. 2003). Remission was nearly twice as likely in individuals receiving treatment at high levels of intensity, defined as at least 8 weeks with no or only minimal symptoms, compared with those that received no treatment, after controlling for propensity for treatment intensity. Although low and moderate levels of treatment did not significantly differ from no treatment, each level of treatment intensity had higher adjusted levels of remission but with overlapping confidence intervals (CIs). In this observational study, intervals receiving higher doses of antidepressants were more likely to achieve remission in this broadly generalizable sample.

In October 2004, the U.S. Food and Drug Administration (FDA) issued a black-box warning to the labeling of all antidepressants used in pediatric patients because of the possibility of increased suicidality. In December 2006, this was extended to young adults after consideration of the risk of suicidal ideation and suicide attempts among participants of hundreds of trials of antidepressants (Leon 2007b). More than two-thirds of the events involved only suicidal ideation. Separate analysis found a significant elevation in risk of suicidal ideation or behavior in children and adolescents and a marginal yet non-significant increase in those ages 18–25 years, whereas those age 65 or older had a significant protective effect (Leon 2007b). These findings generated considerable controversy and were not confirmed on meta-analysis of trial data for suicides (Khan et al. 2003). This black-box warning subsequently led to a marked reduction in antidepressant prescriptions in what some called a large-scale "public health experiment" (Leon 2007a). Indeed, analyses of national data suggested that the decreases in antidepressant prescriptions were accompanied by an uptick in rates of suicide among children and adolescents (Gibbons et al. 2007). Further study of this important issue was clearly warranted.

To address this issue in the CDS data set, Leon et al. (2011) identified 757 participants with unipolar major depression or bipolar disorder. During up to 27 years of follow-up, a total of 6,716 treatment exposure intervals were observed, of which approximately half were associated with antidepressant exposure (3,283) and 3,433 intervals were not. The propensity to receive antidepressants was strongly related to the severity of mood symptoms as well as to a worsening trajectory of severity of symptoms in the preceding 8 weeks. These data on clinical severity and course were used for the development of a propensity score. The mixed-effects, grouped-time survival analyses were stratified by propensity score quintile (to match groups by likelihood of receiving antidepressants), and the results were pooled in the absence of a propensity-by-treatment interaction, which would necessitate reporting of the results by each quintile. The results showed antidepressants to be protective against suicidal behavior (defined as suicide attempts or deaths) in that they appeared to reduce the risk of suicidal behavior by 20% (hazard ratio [HR] = 0.80; 95% CI = 0.68–0.95; $z = -2.54$; $P = 0.01$) (Leon et al. 2011). In this more generalizable sample, and by focusing on actual suicidal behavior and not simply suicidal ideation, there did not appear to be any apparent harm from antidepressant treatment. Rather, antidepressants appeared to have a protective effect, indicated by a 20% reduction in suicidal behavior when methods that account for severity and trajectory of mood symptoms were used.

Some speculated that the protective effect may have been limited to unipolar major depression and questioned the failure to stratify the prior analysis (Leon et al. 2011) by polarity (unipolar vs. bipolar) (Goldberg 2011). Beyond the potential for differential treatment response and risk, this stratification is noteworthy given that FDA meta-analyses suggested greater risk with antidepressants among children and adolescents, and this age group is more likely to progress from unipolar major depression to bipolar disorder (Fiedorowicz et al. 2011). A subsequent analysis included 206 participants with bipolar I disorder (980 treatment intervals exposed to antidepressant and 1,030 treatment intervals unexposed), 139 participants with bipolar II disorder (694 treatment intervals exposed to antidepressants, 713 unexposed intervals), and 361 participants with unipolar major depression (1,417 treatment intervals exposed, 1,328 unexposed intervals) (A.C. Leon, D.A. Solomon, C. Li, et al., unpublished data, January 2013). Treatment intervals did not consider concomitant medications (e.g., antidepressant use as monotherapy vs. part of combination therapy with mood stabilizers for bipolar depression). When similar methods were used to address propensity through matching, mixed-effects, grouped-time survival models unexpectedly found a risk reduction for suicidal behavior by 54% in those with bipolar I disorder (HR=0.46; 95% CI=0.31–0.69; t=–3.74; $P<0.001$) and 35% for those with bipolar II disorder (HR=0.65; 95% CI=0.43–0.99; t=–2.01; $P<0.05$). No evidence of any change in risk of suicidal behavior with antidepressant treatment was seen among those with unipolar major depression in this analysis (HR=0.88; 95% CI=0.64–1.22; t=–0.76; P=0.45) (A.C. Leon, D.A. Solomon, C. Li, et al., unpublished data, January 2013) (Figure 9–1). These unexpected results challenge the burgeoning perception that antidepressants provide no benefit and may be more harmful in bipolar disorder (Goldberg 2012), but caution must be exercised in interpreting these findings. A unipolar versus bipolar polarity-by-exposure interaction was not tested and, in fact, could not be tested, as separate models were developed for each diagnosis. Additionally, the study may have been underpowered to detect such an interaction (Leon and Heo 2009). Thus, although the apparent benefit of antidepressants was significant only for subgroups with bipolar disorder, we cannot conclude that antidepressants provide greater protection for bipolar disorder than for unipolar disorder. Further study is warranted to clarify this relation.

Anticonvulsant Safety

The U.S. FDA similarly warned providers about an elevated risk of suicidal ideation and behavior with antiepileptic drugs, although no black-box warning label was required (U.S. Food and Drug Administration 2009). This action was based on data from 199 randomized clinical trials for a variety of indications, in which 0.37% of individuals taking an antiepileptic drug and 0.24% taking placebo had suicidal ideation or behavior, two-thirds of which was suicidal ideation. Leon et al. (2012) used the CDS data to examine the risk of suicide attempts or deaths related to use of anticonvulsant drugs in a broadly generalizable sample of individuals with bipolar disorder. The analysis used data after 2 years of follow-up because anticonvulsant drugs had not been used in the first 2 years of CDS follow-up. From a sample of 199 CDS participants with bipolar I disorder, 1,077 intervals were defined as exposed (216) or unexposed (861) to the FDA-approved anticonvulsants for bipolar disorder: carbamazepine, lamotrigine, or valproic acid derivatives. This sample included many individuals who would not likely have been included in randomized clinical trials

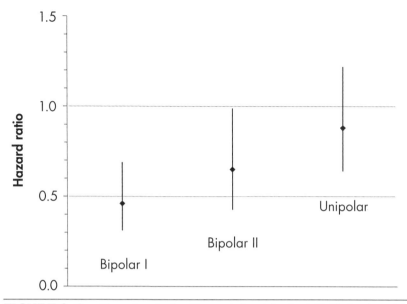

FIGURE 9–1.   Hazard ratios by diagnosis for risk of suicidal behavior with antidepressants.

Note.   This figure provides the estimates for the risk of suicidal behavior (attempts or deaths) in the setting of antidepressants in mood disorders by diagnosis, accounting for the propensity of receiving such treatment. The figure provides the estimates and 95% confidence intervals for hazard ratios derived from mixed-effects, grouped-time survival models. The previously reported protective benefit was significant for bipolar disorder (types I and II) but not for unipolar disorder.

because 9% had made a suicide attempt in the preceding 3 months, 33% were at most mildly symptomatic at onset of the relevant exposure interval, and 15% had psychotic symptoms or extreme functional impairment. Propensity to receive anticonvulsants was strongly related to severe manic symptoms or hypomanic symptoms and inversely related to use of antipsychotics, which presumably were alternatively, instead of additionally, prescribed to target such symptoms. Because of sparse strata, rather than stratification by quintile of propensity score, an optimal matching procedure was used. The unadjusted rates of suicidal behavior or deaths were 6.3% for unexposed and 5.1% for exposed intervals. In the matched set of 852 intervals, mixed-effects, grouped-time survival models indicated no increased risk of suicidal behavior related to anticonvulsant exposure (HR=0.93; 95% CI=0.45–1.92; $z=-0.2$; $P=0.8$). A sensitivity analysis using a less stringent matching criterion and including 1,063 of the intervals had similar results (HR=0.87; 95% CI=0.42–1.79; $z=-0.4$; $P=0.4$). Thus, over the long-term follow-up of the broadly generalizable CDS sample, there did not appear to be any increased risk of suicidal behavior associated with anticonvulsant use. This suggests that the findings largely related to suicidal ideation in short-term trials may not generalize to clinical practice, although regular monitoring and safety assessments of individuals with bipolar disorder treated with anticonvulsants are certainly indicated.

Conclusion

Over several decades of its history, the CDS proved to be a valuable resource in examining the safety and effectiveness of somatic therapies for mood disorders, and the work has shown that observational data may prove useful for a variety of clinically relevant questions. These existing observational data have importantly been able to weigh in on clinical controversies relatively quickly without the need for a new study. This may be useful for clarifying questions that were not considered prior to study design, as well as for directing the design of subsequent studies. Prudent use of observational data for questions related to the effectiveness and safety of treatments, however, requires rigorous methods to address issues of confounding and the propensity to receive specific therapies. The CDS data have determined that clinical variables related to severity and course of illness in mood disorders are highly relevant to this propensity. This information is also relevant to studies that estimate propensity from samples lacking the relevant data for such determination.

Clinical Implications

- Antidepressants are effective at higher doses for the treatment of acute episodes of major depression, even in broader samples than those represented in clinical trials.
- Antidepressants are effective in preventing recurrence following remission of major depressive disorder and should be maintained at the full dose required to achieve remission.
- When the clinical features affecting propensity to receive treatment are taken into account, antidepressants and antiepileptic medications do not appear to increase the risk of suicidal behavior. Antidepressants even had a protective effect in the Collaborative Depression Study cohort. Close monitoring for risk of suicide is indicated for individuals receiving treatment for mood disorders, given the associated risk.

References

Coryell W, Winokur G, Solomon D, et al: Lithium and recurrence in a long-term follow-up of bipolar affective disorder. Psychol Med 27:281–289, 1997

Coryell W, Solomon D, Leon AC, et al: Lithium discontinuation and subsequent effectiveness. Am J Psychiatry 155:895–898, 1998

Dawson R, Lavori PW, Coryell WH, et al: Maintenance strategies for unipolar depression: an observational study of levels of treatment and recurrence. J Affect Disord 49:31–44, 1998

Fiedorowicz JG, Endicott J, Leon AC, et al: Subthreshold hypomanic symptoms in progression from unipolar major depression to bipolar disorder. Am J Psychiatry 168:40–48, 2011

Frank E, Kupfer DJ, Perel JM, et al: Three-year outcomes for maintenance therapies in recurrent depression. Arch Gen Psychiatry 47:1093–1099, 1990

Geddes JR, Carney SM, Davies C, et al: Relapse prevention with antidepressant drug treatment in depressive disorders: a systematic review. Lancet 361:653–661, 2003

Gelenberg AJ, Kane JM, Keller MB, et al: Comparison of standard and low serum levels of lithium for maintenance treatment of bipolar disorder. N Engl J Med 321:1489–1493, 1989

Gibbons RD, Brown CH, Hur K, et al: Early evidence on the effects of regulators' suicidality warnings on SSRI prescriptions and suicide in children and adolescents. Am J Psychiatry 164:1356–1363, 2007

Goldberg JF: Antidepressant use and risk for suicide attempts in bipolar disorder. J Clin Psychiatry 72:1697; author reply 1697, 2011

Goldberg JF: Antidepressants: the scapegoat of poor outcome bipolar disorder? Aust N Z J Psychiatry 46:302–305, 2012

Keller MB, Lavori PW, Mueller TI, et al: Time to recovery, chronicity, and levels of psychopathology in major depression: a 5-year prospective follow-up of 431 subjects. Arch Gen Psychiatry 49:809–816, 1992

Khan A, Khan S, Kolts R, et al: Suicide rates in clinical trials of SSRIs, other antidepressants, and placebo: analysis of FDA reports. Am J Psychiatry 160:790–792, 2003

Kupfer DJ, Frank E, Perel JM, et al: Five-year outcome for maintenance therapies in recurrent depression. Arch Gen Psychiatry 49:769–773, 1992

Lavori PW, Keller MB, Mueller TI, et al: Recurrence after recovery in unipolar MDD: an observational follow-up study of clinical predictors and somatic treatment as a mediating factor. Int J Methods Psychiatr Res 4:211–229, 1994

Leon AC: The revised black box warning for antidepressants sets a public health experiment in motion. J Clin Psychiatry 68:1139–1141, 2007a

Leon AC: The revised warning for antidepressants and suicidality: unveiling the black box of statistical analyses. Am J Psychiatry 164:1786–1789, 2007b

Leon AC, Hedeker D: A mixed-effects quintile-stratified propensity adjustment for effectiveness analyses of ordered categorical doses. Stat Med 24:647–658, 2005

Leon AC, Heo M: Sample sizes required to detect interactions between two binary fixed-effects in a mixed-effects linear regression model. Comput Stat Data Anal 53:603–608, 2009

Leon AC, Mueller TI, Solomon DA, et al: A dynamic adaptation of the propensity score adjustment for effectiveness analyses of ordinal doses of treatment. Stat Med 20:1487–1498, 2001

Leon AC, Solomon DA, Mueller TI, et al: A 20-year longitudinal observational study of somatic antidepressant treatment effectiveness. Am J Psychiatry 160:727–733, 2003

Leon AC, Solomon DA, Li C, et al: Antidepressants and risks of suicide and suicide attempts: a 27-year observational study. J Clin Psychiatry 72:580–586, 2011

Leon AC, Solomon DA, Li C, et al: Antiepileptic drugs for bipolar disorder and the risk of suicidal behavior: a 30-year observational study. Am J Psychiatry 169:285–291, 2012

Prabhakar M, Haynes WG, Coryell WH, et al: Factors associated with the prescribing of olanzapine, quetiapine, and risperidone in patients with bipolar and related affective disorders. Pharmacotherapy 31:806–812, 2011

Prien RF, Kupfer DJ, Mansky PA, et al: Drug therapy in the prevention of recurrences in unipolar and bipolar affective disorders: report of the NIMH Collaborative Study Group comparing lithium carbonate, imipramine, and a lithium carbonate-imipramine combination. Arch Gen Psychiatry 41:1096–1104, 1984

Robinson DS, Lerfald SC, Bennett B, et al: Continuation and maintenance treatment of major depression with the monoamine oxidase inhibitor phenelzine: a double-blind placebo-controlled discontinuation study. Psychopharmacol Bull 27:31–39, 1991

Solomon DA, Leon AC, Mueller TI, et al: Tachyphylaxis in unipolar major depressive disorder. J Clin Psychiatry 66:283–290, 2005

Tondo L, Baldessarini RJ, Floris G, et al: Effectiveness of restarting lithium treatment after its discontinuation in bipolar I and bipolar II disorders. Am J Psychiatry 154:548–550, 1997

U.S. Food and Drug Administration: Suicidal behavior and ideation and antiepileptic drugs. May 5, 2009. Available at: http://www.fda.gov/Drugs/DrugSafety/PostmarketDrugSafetyInformationforPatientsandProviders/ucm100190.htm. Accessed May 19, 2012.

CHAPTER 10

Personality and Mood Disorders

Robert M.A. Hirschfeld, M.D.

VARIOUS RELATIONS between personality and depression have been described for several thousand years. This long and rich history was based on clinical observation, leading to development of diverse theories. Hippocrates believed that depression arose from a premorbid temperament of melancholia caused by an excess of black bile, one of the body's four basic humors (Adams 1939). This formulation endured for centuries, as illustrated by the German psychiatrist Kretschmer's belief that "endogenous psychoses are nothing other than marked accentuation of normal types of temperament" (Kretschmer 1936; quoted in Akiskal et al. 1983). Psychoanalytic theory continued this approach, regarding psychopathological states as arising from predisposing personality traits (Akiskal et al. 1983; Arieti and Bemporad 1978). When the National Institute of Mental Health Collaborative Depression Study (CDS) began, relatively little objective, reproducible research had been done to test these and other theories of the relation between personality and depression. The CDS provided an outstanding opportunity to gather empirical data to support such research.

Ways in Which Personality and Depression May Relate

The nature of this relation between personality and depression may be conceptualized in several alternative, but not mutually exclusive, ways (Hirschfeld 1986).

The *predispositional (or vulnerability) approach* has predominated historically in both theory and research, as noted earlier. This view proposes that particular personality characteristics are antecedent to depressive disorders and render the person possessing them vulnerable to depression under certain conditions.

At the time of the design of the CDS, the most widely held view with regard to the predispositional approach was that undue interpersonal dependency predisposed individuals to depression (Hirschfeld et al. 1976). *Interpersonal dependency* referred to a complex of thoughts, beliefs, feelings, and behaviors revolving around needs to associate closely with valued other people. It was based conceptually on psychoanalytic theory, social learning theories of dependency, and the ethological theory of attachment (Hirschfeld et al. 1976). Key to this issue was emotional reliance on another person and lack of social self-confidence. Depression was thought to result when an individual with excessive amounts of interpersonal dependency had that dependency thwarted in some way. Prior to the CDS, no empirical measure of interpersonal dependency had existed, so members of the CDS team developed a 48-item self-report inventory (Hirschfeld et al. 1977).

The *complication approach* is the opposite of the predispositional approach. According to the complication approach, one consequence of the experience of a clinical depression is personality change, particularly when the episode is severe and protracted. Thus, the subjective, devastating experience of a depression may lead to and cause changes in personality in terms of an individual's perception of himself or herself and his or her style of interacting with other people. Furthermore, depression and its resulting personality changes may lead others to treat the depressed individual differently, resulting in further changes. For example, pessimism and dependency may become permanent features of personality following multiple depressive episodes.

The *subclinical approach* focuses on the relation between temperamental, or constitutionally based, aspects of personality and affective disorders (Hirschfeld and Klerman 1979; Widiger and Trull 1992). According to this view, whose proponents include Kraepelin, Kretschmer, and Akiskal, certain personality characteristics may be considered milder manifestations of affective disorders, with both representing expressions of the same underlying genetic endowment. Thus, certain behavior patterns, such as cyclothymia, are viewed as part of a continuum blending at one end with normality and at the other with a depressive or hypomanic episode.

The *pathoplasty model* proposes that personality characteristics influence the symptomatic expression and course of the depressive episode but are not etiological or involved in the pathogenesis of depression. Thus, certain personality types may be associated with specific depressive symptom profiles, such as a histrionic personality with more hostile, angry, complaining symptoms during the depressive episode (Hirschfeld and Klerman 1979; Widiger and Trull 1992).

The State/Trait Issue

Before being able to assess the ways that personality and depression may relate, we had to address whether standard assessment techniques measured true personality traits or traits altered by the clinical state of depression. That is, the presence of being clinically depressed may alter the assessment of personality traits. In fact, this could have inadvertently influenced clinical theorists because, in general, clinicians see patients more often during an episode of illness than when they are well. Clinical observation and the resulting perception may be of a personality altered by the clinical state.

CDS investigators used several strategies to address this issue. Each patient was asked to answer questions according to his or her "usual self"—that is, his or her typical way of acting or feeling during asymptomatic periods. This request was made to minimize the effect of illness on response, a technique that had been used successfully in other studies. The personality inventories were administered to inpatients near the time of hospital discharge when symptomatology had improved substantially (Hirschfeld and Klerman 1979). We used these instructions with 73 patients with depression and compared these results with the published norms. Depressed patients were found to be significantly more neurotic and introverted than the published norms for these scales.

The personality battery was readministered to the same patients at their 1-year follow-up evaluation. We then were able to compare the scores of patients in remission or recovery (i.e., with no more than minimal symptoms of the index episode for at least 8 consecutive weeks) with scores obtained from the same subjects at the initial evaluation. We found substantial changes in personality between the entry evaluation and the follow-up in these recovered patients (Hirschfeld et al. 1983). This outcome was particularly true for measures of emotional strength and interpersonal dependency. Scores made when patients had fully recovered reflected a much "healthier" personality in terms of less neuroticism, orality, and emotional reliance on another person and more ego resiliency and social self-confidence. In addition, patients had an increase in extroversion and sociability when well at the 1-year follow-up. Interestingly, patients who had not recovered at the time of the 1-year follow-up had no significant changes in personality assessment from their entry scores. This outcome strongly suggests that assessment of these personality features is very much influenced by clinical state.

Personality Change and Depression

Shea and associates (1996) examined whether personality traits change after an episode of depression. Subjects with a prospectively observed first episode of major depression were compared with subjects who remained well over a 6-year interval. No evidence of a negative change in personality was found from pre- to postmorbid assessment of personality.

Premorbid Personality Traits and Depression

The best test of the personality-depression relation would involve assessment of personality *before* the onset of the first depressive episode, and the CDS afforded us that opportunity with our sample of relatives, spouses, and control subjects. Twenty-nine subjects from our sample of relatives, spouses, and control subjects with no history of mental disorder subsequently had a first onset of major depression (Hirschfeld et al. 1989). We were able to compare the intake personality qualities of these 29 subjects with those of 370 subjects who continued to be free of illness during the 6-year follow-up period. Those who became ill had significantly higher neuroticism and decreased emotional stability than did those who did not become ill.

Somewhat to our surprise, we did not find a significant difference in measures of interpersonal dependency between these two groups or differences in extroversion or sociability. When the sample was divided into those whose first major depressive episode began earlier or later than age 30, the differences in neuroticism and emotional strength occurred only in the older first-onset group. Among subjects whose onset of illness was between ages 17 and 30 years, no differences in personality variables were seen between the two groups.

We concluded that there was not support for a specific personality feature of undue interpersonal dependency in the onset of unipolar depression. We did find support for a role of nonspecific personality features of neuroticism and decreased emotional strength in the onset of unipolar depression after age 30. We also found that personality assessment is strongly influenced by clinical state, suggesting that clinical assessments of personality conducted while patients are depressed may reflect their clinical state rather than (or in addition to) enduring personality traits.

Personality and Bipolarity

We also investigated the relation of personality to polarity (Hirschfeld et al. 1986). In this analysis, we compared the personality traits of 45 patients with bipolar disorder who were fully recovered with those of 78 patients with unipolar depression who also had recovered, as well as with those of 1,172 never mentally ill first-degree relatives of our patients. Very few differences were found between the recovered bipolar patients and recovered unipolar patients. No differences were seen between female unipolar and bipolar patients. Among males, the only significant differences between the groups were increased general activity and ascendance (measures of submissiveness and hesitancy). However, significant differences were found between the two depressed groups and the never-ill comparison groups on all issues of emotional strength and on interpersonal dependency. These findings suggest that individuals with depression, regardless of polarity, can be distinguished from those who never become ill.

A subsequent analysis of the same data focused on individual item differences rather than scale differences. Bipolar I patients were seen as more normal in terms of emotional stability and extroversion. Bipolar II patients were described as more neurotic, labile, energetic, assertive, sensitive, and brooding (Akiskal et al. 2006).

Clinical Implications

- Clinical evaluations of personality conducted when patients are depressed may lead to inaccurate conclusions. Depressed patients view themselves as being more neurotic, less resilient, more interpersonally dependent, and less self-confident than after they have recovered from their depression.
- Individuals who are more neurotic and less emotionally strong are more likely to become depressed than are those who are not. These personality features are probably nonspecific and may predict other psychiatric illnesses as well.
- Individuals who are highly emotionally dependent on another person are not necessarily more likely to become depressed than are those who are not as emotionally dependent.

References

Adams F (ed): The Genuine Works of Hippocrates. Baltimore, MD, Williams & Wilkins, 1939

Akiskal HS, Hirschfeld RMA, Yerevanian BI: The relationship of personality to affective disorders. Arch Gen Psychiatry 40:801–810, 1983

Akiskal HS, Kilzieh N, Maser JD, et al: The distinct temperament profiles of bipolar I, bipolar II and unipolar patients. J Affect Disord 92:19–33, 2006

Arieti S, Bemporad J: Severe and Mild Depression. New York, Basic Books, 1978

Hirschfeld RMA: Personality and bipolar disorder, in Results in Depression Research. Edited by Hippius H, Klerman GL, Matussek N. Heidelberg, Germany, Springer-Verlag, 1986

Hirschfeld RMA, Klerman GL: Personality attributes and affective disorders. Am J Psychiatry 136:67–70, 1979

Hirschfeld RMA, Klerman GL, Chodoff P, et al: Dependency-self-esteem-clinical depression. J Am Acad Psychoanal 4:373–388, 1976

Hirschfeld RMA, Klerman GL, Gough HG, et al: A measure of interpersonal dependency. J Pers Assess 41:610–618, 1977

Hirschfeld RMA, Klerman GL, Clayton PJ, et al: Assessing personality: effects of depressive state on trait measurement. Am J Psychiatry 140:695–699, 1983

Hirschfeld RMA, Klerman GL, Keller MB, et al: Personality of recovered patients with bipolar affective disorder. J Affect Disord 11:81–89, 1986

Hirschfeld RMA, Klerman GL, Lavori P, et al: Premorbid personality assessments of first onset of major depression. Arch Gen Psychiatry 46:345–350, 1989

Kretschmer E: Physique and Character. Translated by Miller E. London, England, Kegan Paul, Trench, Trubner, 1936

Shea MT, Leon AC, Mueller TI, et al: Does major depression result in lasting personality change? Am J Psychiatry 153:1404–1410, 1996

Widiger TA, Trull TJ: Personality and psychopathology: an application of the five-factor model. J Pers 60:363–393, 1992

CHAPTER 11

Family History and Genetic Studies in Mood Disorders

John P. Rice, Ph.D.

ROBINS AND GUZE, in 1970, delineated five phases for establishing diagnostic validity: clinical description, laboratory studies, delimitation from other diagnoses, follow-up, and family studies. Since then, the wide acceptance of structured diagnostic interviews and complex, comprehensive diagnostic schemata has led to systematic progress. With the introduction of structured interviews, it became necessary to validate a particular instrument and the underlying diagnostic constructs. The Collaborative Depression Study (CDS) followed this tradition established by the Robins and Guze criteria for validation. We performed test-retest studies of the Lifetime Version of the Schedule for Affective Disorders and Schizophrenia (SADS-L; Endicott and Spitzer 1978) early in the CDS, and we used indices of rater agreement to determine psychometric properties and to ensure uniformity among raters. In addition, we compared diagnoses made with direct interview with those made with the family history method (Andreasen et al. 1986) in our sample of relatives. These studies confirmed the usefulness of the family history method, and these procedures that used interview, family history, and best estimate diagnoses were later adapted for the large-scale genetic studies begun in the 1990s.

Relatives of CDS probands were interviewed between 1978 and 1982. Initial analyses focused on rates of illness in the relatives. The most striking finding was the detection of a strong secular trend for major depressive disorder (MDD), with more recently born individuals at increased risk (Klerman et al. 1985).

The second level of analysis was to cross-classify the rates in relatives by the diagnosis of the proband. These analyses showed that the affective disorders are familial and, moreover, that there is specificity by major subtype. That is, relatives of bipolar probands have a higher rate of bipolar disorder than do the relatives of MDD probands. Interestingly, schizoaffective disorder, manic subtype, appeared to segregate with bipolar I disorder, whereas the depressive subtype did not. In many current genetic studies, bipolar I disorder and schizoaffective disorder, manic subtype, are combined in analysis, whereas schizoaffective disorder, depressive subtype, subjects are excluded.

As part of the CDS, a second, blind reassessment of all relatives was performed 6 years after their initial assessment. Of those positive for MDD at initial evaluation, 74% were positive at follow-up (i.e., were also given a lifetime MDD diagnosis by the blind rater 6 years later). There was a gradient: 48% of those who had three symptoms and no treatment received a consistent assessment at follow-up, compared with 96% of those with eight symptoms and treatment who received a diagnosis of MDD at the second assessment. For MDD, we developed a caseness index that predicted diagnostic stability over time. In addition, a hierarchical analysis indicated that bipolar I disorder tends to be diagnosed as schizoaffective disorder, manic subtype, across occasions and vice versa. This analysis is consistent with the prior familial analyses that suggested these two diagnoses be combined into a single bipolar phenotype. In contrast, the analysis for MDD indicates that caseness appears to represent quantitative rather than qualitative differences, with no natural cutoff to identify distinct subgroups. I describe these analyses in the section "Stability of Diagnosis" below.

Results

Secular Trends in Major Depressive Disorder

Variations in rates of illness over time (secular trends) are well established for many medical conditions, including the major mental illnesses. Most disorders, other than congenital defects, have an age effect in that the rate of illness increases as a birth cohort of individuals becomes older. Accordingly, genetic and family studies traditionally have compared the lifetime morbid risk in the population with that in classes of relatives of affected individuals (Slater and Cowie 1971), whereas age-specific rates usually are reported in epidemiological studies. The use of lifetime prevalence can be problematic when secular trends are also present, such that rates in younger individuals already exceed lifetime morbid risks in older individuals.

In addition to age effects, one can consider (birth) cohort effects, in which rates of illness at each age are influenced by factors that depend on the cohort of birth. The size of one's birth cohort (e.g., the "baby boomers") provides an example. In a birth cohort effect, rates depend on the year of birth, whereas in a period effect, the calendar year, which cuts across different cohorts at different ages, is a key variable. Events such as war, radiation exposure (e.g., the recent nuclear reactor meltdown in Japan), or drug availability in the late 1960s are examples of period effects. Note that such effects typically interact with age. For example, drug availability might have had a significant effect on those who were young in the 1960s but a minor effect on those who were older at the time of exposure. Age, cohort, and period are linearly confounded; for example, if one knows a person was age 20 in 2000, one knows that he or she was born in 1980. In general, given any two values, the third can be determined, so that if all three quantities are predictor variables in a linear model, the parameters of the model cannot be estimated. That is, multiple combinations of the three effects would describe the same data. Although statistical analysis alone cannot decide between alternative models, other criteria such as parsimony may be used (Fienberg and Mason 1979).

Several studies of major depression conducted at the same time as the CDS reported strong secular trends (the Epidemiologic Catchment Area Study, Robins et al. 1984; the Camberwell Registry Study, Sturt et al. 1984) with the frequency of lifetime depression lowest in older cohorts and increasing in more recent cohorts. Klerman and colleagues (1985) used life-table methods with 2,289 relatives from the CDS to examine rates of MDD. Figures 11–1 and 11–2 depict the cumulative probability of MDD for male and female relatives, respectively.

Increasing rates of MDD were experienced by successive birth cohorts. These effects were significant ($P < 0.001$) when tested with the Cox proportional hazards regression model. The magnitude of the male-female difference varied across cohorts, with lesser differences for more recently born individuals (Rice et al. 1984). We examined the results for possible artifacts such as memory effects or differential mortality but concluded that they were not due to the possible artifacts examined.

In a later analysis (Lavori et al. 1993), we performed bivariate survival analysis of the initial and 6-year follow-up diagnoses and examined strata defined by several environmental variables. The cohort trend existed in all strata with nearly uniform linearity.

Familial Transmission

As part of the CDS, data were collected on 2,225 first-degree relatives of 612 probands. We analyzed (Rice et al. 1987b) 187 families of bipolar patients

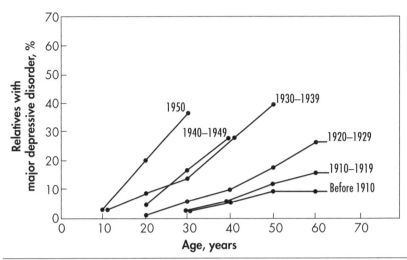

FIGURE 11–1. Cumulative probability of diagnosable major depressive disorder in male relatives by birth cohort.

Source. Adapted from Klerman et al. 1985.

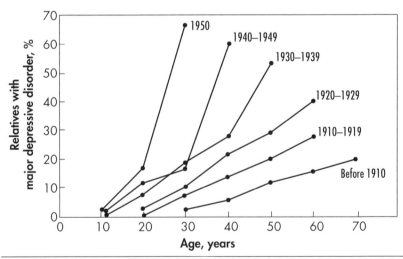

FIGURE 11–2. Cumulative probability of diagnosable major depressive disorder in female relatives by birth cohort.

Source. Adapted from Klerman et al. 1985.

(149 probands with a diagnosis of bipolar I disorder and 38 with a diagnosis of schizoaffective disorder, manic subtype). We used traditional genetic methods and found that the morbid risk of bipolar illness was 5.7% in the relatives of bipolar probands as contrasted with 1.1% in the relatives of probands with major depression. These values compared closely with those obtained with survival analysis. Relatives of probands with early age at onset were found to have a greater risk than were relatives of probands with late onset. The sex of the relative, the sex of the proband, or the subtype of the proband (bipolar I or schizoaffective bipolar) did not influence the risk in the relative. The age at onset was accelerated within birth cohorts, with individuals born in more recent cohorts having an earlier onset.

A hierarchical lifetime diagnosis was created according to the following order (highest precedence to lowest): schizophrenia; schizoaffective disorder, manic subtype; schizoaffective disorder, depressive subtype only; bipolar I disorder; bipolar II disorder; and MDD. Individuals with a diagnosis of schizoaffective disorder, manic subtype, and individuals with diagnoses of both schizoaffective disorder, depressive subtype, and bipolar I disorder were included as having schizoaffective disorder, manic subtype. Individuals with a diagnosis of mania (or hypomania) without an additional diagnosis of major, minor, or intermittent depression were classified as having bipolar I disorder (or bipolar II disorder). The probands and relatives are cross-classified by this hierarchical diagnosis in Table 11–1. We evaluated the hypothesis of Gershon and colleagues (1982) that schizoaffective disorder lies on a continuum with bipolar I disorder. We noted that the (not age-corrected) rates of bipolar I disorder were the highest in the relatives of the probands with schizoaffective disorder, manic subtype, and bipolar I disorder. We noted, moreover, that the rate of schizophrenia was elevated in the relatives of probands with schizoaffective disorder, depressive subtype, when compared with the relatives of probands with MDD ($P < 0.001$) but not in the relatives of probands with schizoaffective disorder, manic subtype. After examining the data of Gershon and colleagues, we found rates of schizophrenia of 3.6% compared with 0% in the relatives of their schizoaffective and control probands ($P < 0.06$, Fisher exact test).

Accordingly, we retained for analysis only the families in which the proband had a hierarchical diagnosis of schizoaffective disorder, manic subtype, or bipolar I disorder. The rates of illness in the 187 bipolar families are given in Table 11–2, along with rates in the relatives of the 331 probands with MDD (without a lifetime diagnosis of schizoaffective illness, mania, or hypomania). We used survival analysis to test the significance of several variables on the rates shown in Table 11–2.

We found that the proband's age at onset was significantly related to the risk of illness in the relatives ($P < 0.005$)—probands with an earlier onset im-

TABLE 11–1. Hierarchical diagnosis in interviewed relatives: Collaborative Depression Study

	Proband's diagnosis					
	SA/M	**SA/D**	**BP-I**	**BP-II**	**MDD**	**Total**
No. of families	38	16	149	78	331	612
No. of relatives	139	72	567	271	1,176	2,225
Relative's diagnosis (%)						
Schizophrenia	0.7	2.8	1.1	0.4	0.3	...
SA/M	0.7	0.0	0.5	0.4	0.2	...
SA/D	0.0	0.0	0.2	0.0	0.3	...
BP-I	3.6	0.0	3.9	1.1	0.6	...
BP-II	5.8	6.9	6.5	10.0	4.8	...
MDD	23.0	22.2	23.1	26.9	28.6	...

Note. BP-I and BP-II=bipolar I and II disorder; MDD=major depressive disorder; SA/M=schizoaffective disorder, manic subtype; SA/D=schizoaffective disorder, depressive subtype.

TABLE 11–2. Rates of bipolar illness in relatives classified by relationship to proband

	Proband no. (%)[a]			
	Interview data		Family history data	
Relationship	**Bipolar** (*n*=187)	**Major depression** (*n*=331)	**Bipolar** (*n*=187)	**Major depression** (*n*=331)
Father	6.4 (5/78)	0.0 (0/160)	6.5 (12/186)	2.1 (7/331)
Mother	4.1 (5/121)	1.0 (2/197)	6.4 (12/187)	1.5 (5/330)
Brother	6.0(10/168)	1.1 (3/267)	6.0 (15/252)	1.1 (5/460)
Sister	4.3 (9/209)	0.9 (3/352)	6.0 (16/266)	0.6 (3/473)
Son	1.6 (1/62)	0.0 (0/100)	3.6 (3/83)	0.8 (1/133)
Daughter	1.5 (1/68)	0.8 (1/130)	5.1 (4/78)	0.7 (1/152)
Spouse	0.0 (0/72)	0.0 (0/149)	2.4 (3/123)	0.7 (2/282)

[a]Interview data based on Schedule for Affective Disorders and Schizophrenia–Lifetime Version; family history based on Family History Research Diagnostic Criteria, obtained from proband and best informant.

parted greater risk. In addition, the effect of the relative's birth cohort was significant ($P < 0.01$), paralleling a similar finding for unipolar illness in our data (Klerman et al. 1985).

Stability of Diagnosis

Studies of reliability have used either joint or separate evaluations spaced a few days, weeks, or months apart to quantify rater agreement. Reliability results are usually quantified in terms of the κ statistic. Difficulties are associated with κ because it has a strong dependence on the base rate in the population being sampled. These issues may be more important for the assessment of nonpatients (e.g., relatives of patients or a general population sample). A concept related to test-retest reliability is that of temporal stability, wherein interviews are given at widely separated points in time or at successive hospital admissions. Although both paradigms use independent evaluations at two times, emphases and assumptions differ, and we use the term *stability* rather than *long-term reliability* to indicate this.

A situation in which a subject is positive for a lifetime diagnosis at index evaluation and then negative for that lifetime diagnosis at follow-up represents a diagnostic error. We use those positive at index to quantify and model this error. A related goal is to be able to redefine who is considered a case. For example, we defined a quantitative scale (based on certainty of diagnosis) for each subject with a diagnosis of MDD. This requires the distinction between the observed state and the true state, of which we have imperfect measures.

Sensitivity, Specificity, and True Case Rate

A model that is widely used in evaluating screening tests when the true state can be determined is defined in terms of the sensitivity p (the probability of correctly diagnosing a true case) and the specificity q (the probability of correctly diagnosing a true noncase). The observed prevalence is the sum of the rate of true cases that are correctly diagnosed and the rate of noncases that are incorrectly diagnosed (false positives). In the context of a reliability study, Kraemer (1979) related p, q, and true base rate K with the value of κ from a test-retest reliability study. She noted the interdependence between the value of κ and the true base rate when the sensitivity and specificity were constant across populations.

Use of Clinical Predictors

We then considered a set of predictors for an observed case at time 1. The variables may include the number of symptoms, treatment-seeking behavior, and sex, as indicated in Table 11–3. We found a gradient: 48% of those who had three symptoms and no treatment received a consistent assessment at follow-up, compared with 96% of those with eight symptoms and treatment who received a diagnosis of MDD at the second assessment. Following the methods outlined in our prior work (Rice et al. 1987a, 1992), we used a logistic model to predict who would be positive at time 2 among those who were positive at time 1. We further assumed that all observed cases were true cases at the highest possible covariate value, Z_{max}, so that the sensitivity could be estimated. Moreover, we could then derive the probability of being a true case at time 2, conditioned on being positive at time 1. Accordingly, we could use values of variables such as number of depressive symptoms, number of episodes, and treatment-seeking behavior to derive a single score to indicate how likely the individual is a true case (as derived from our stability analysis).

In a subsequent analysis (Rice and Todorov 1994), we used the four levels of severity of MDD based on the index of caseness, denoted MDD-A, MDD-B, MDD-C, and MDD-D—these variables represent decreasing levels of caseness. We created six dummy variables corresponding to the seven categories MDD-A, MDD-B, MDD-C, MDD-D, minor depression, other diagnosis, and never mentally ill. The resulting odds ratios for MDD represented a gradient of risk (Table 11–4), with a regression coefficient of 0.65. The resulting odds ratios were similar to those obtained when ordinality of the categories was not assumed. The hypothesis of ordinality is accepted. In contrast to the ordinal relationship for MDD, hypomania in combination with the index of caseness for MDD did not define an ordinal relationship for stability of hypomania. The ordinal model in Table 11–5 gives a χ^2 of 62.0 with four degrees of freedom ($P < 0.001$), whereas the model with an effect of only the presence of hypomania (with or without MDD) gave an odds ratio of 34.3 and a good fit to the data. The predictors of mania are given in Table 11–6. It is interesting that hypomania predicts intermediate odds between mania and MDD across occasions. This extends a prior analysis (Rice et al. 1986) that indicated that despite the low test-retest reliability of bipolar II disorder as measured by κ, it appears to be a useful diagnosis when considered as part of an affective disorder spectrum.

Comments

We found marked secular trends in analyses of alcohol dependence (Rice et al. 2003) similar to those found for MDD in the CDS. The striking result in both studies was the low rate in older individuals, with rates in younger individuals already exceeding those in older cohorts. Thus, without controlling for birth cohort, one might conclude that these conditions are nonfamilial because the rate in parents is lower than the overall prevalence. This finding underscores the need for modeling secular trends when analyzing familial data, whether the effect is real or the result of a methodological artifact. The cohorts with

TABLE 11–3. Stability of lifetime major depressive disorder (MDD) diagnosis over 6 years, by clinical covariates

Covariate	No. of relatives	*n* (%) with stable diagnosis
Major depression	519	383 (74)
No. of symptoms***		
3	49	26 (53)
4	111	69 (62)
5	98	74 (76)
6	112	88 (79)
7	81	65 (80)
8	67	61 (91)
No. of episodes***		
1	292	200 (68)
2	97	75 (77)
3	130	109 (84)
Attempted suicide**		
No	428	305 (71)
Yes	91	79 (87)
Hospitalized***		
No	416	291 (70)
Yes	103	93 (90)
Incapacitated***		
No	449	320 (71)
Yes	70	64 (91)
Received medication***		
No	260	169 (65)
Yes	259	215 (83)
Treated for MDD***		
No	249	160 (64)
Yes	270	224 (83)

TABLE 11–3. Stability of lifetime major depressive disorder (MDD) diagnosis over 6 years, by clinical covariates *(continued)*

Covariate	No. of relatives	n (%) with stable diagnosis
Duration of longest period, weeks*		
2	55	34 (62)
3–4	58	39 (67)
5–51	244	185 (76)
52	154	119 (77)
Sex		
Male	160	113 (71)
Female	359	271 (75)

Note. Patients were treated for MDD, hospitalized, received medication, or received electroconvulsive therapy.
* $P < 0.05$. ** $P < 0.01$. *** $P < 0.001$.

TABLE 11–4. Predictors of lifetime major depressive disorder (MDD) diagnosis at time 2, by lifetime diagnosis at time 1 (6 years earlier)

Time 1 diagnosis	Categorical analysis		Ordinal analysis
	Odds ratio	χ^2	
MDD-A	53.8	141.4	50.2
MDD-B	24.5	102.2	26.1
MDD-C	13.9	101.6	13.6
MDD-D	7.2	90.5	7.1
Minor depression	2.6	14.8	3.7
Other diagnosis	1.9	12.4	1.9
Never mentally ill	1.0	—	1.0

TABLE 11–5. Predictors of lifetime hypomania diagnosis at time 2, by lifetime diagnosis at time 1 (6 years earlier)

Time 1 diagnosis	Odds ratio	χ^2	Effect of hypomania	Ordinal analysis
Hypomania				
MDD-A	45.8	54.5		65.9
MDD-B	27.5	24.3		28.5
MDD-C	39.3	27.2	34.3	12.3
MDD-D	38.2	32.1		5.3
No MDD	26.2	38.8		2.3
MDD	4.2	13.8	4.1	1.6
Minor depression	3.5	5.0	3.5	1.4
Other diagnosis	2.5	3.9	2.5	1.0
Never mentally ill	1.0	—	—	—
Model fit (degrees of freedom)			1.2 (4)	62.0 (4)

Note. MDD = major depressive disorder.

TABLE 11–6. Predictors of lifetime mania diagnosis at time 2, by lifetime diagnosis at time 1 (6 years earlier)

Time 1 diagnosis	Odds ratio	χ^2
Mania	88.2	87.2
Hypomania	15.1	16.9
Major depressive disorder	3.3	5.4
Never mentally ill	1.0	—

the lowest rates of MDD in Figures 11–1 and 11–2 would likely be deceased and not present in studies conducted today, so replication of our study would be problematic.

Apart from some genetic linkage studies (Cox et al. 1989), the CDS did not carry out genetic analyses per se. The CDS did, however, contribute to the design and phenotypic definition of recent genetic studies. Some established association results are now available for bipolar disorder (Psychiatric GWAS Consortium Bipolar Disorder Working Group 2011; Sklar et al. 2008), although the variance explained is quite small. The Psychiatric GWAS Consortium Bipolar Disorder Working Group had more than 7,000 case patients and 9,000 control subjects by combining data from 11 studies. It is not surprising that older, small studies had not been successful in the genetic analysis of bipolar disorder. For MDD, the Major Depressive Disorder Working Group of the Psychiatric GWAS Consortium (2011) analyzed more than 9,000 case patients and 9,000 control subjects in a discovery set and almost 7,000 case patients and more than 50,000 control subjects in a replication set. No consistent signals were detected in replication. Accordingly, although bipolar disorder and MDD have high heritability, it has proven difficult to identify specific susceptibility genes. Perhaps other phenotypic definitions will provide more clinically homogeneous samples for analysis.

Clinical Implications

- Major depressive disorder has a strong secular trend, with more recently born individuals at increased risk. (Lack of consideration of these secular trends in genetic analysis may be problematic.)
- The affective disorders are familial, and moreover, there is specificity by subtype.
- Schizoaffective disorder, manic subtype, appears to be part of the bipolar spectrum, whereas schizoaffective disorder, depressive subtype, does not.
- MDD appears to represent a continuum based on severity, whereas bipolar I disorder appears to be more categorical.
- Despite the low test-retest reliability of bipolar II disorder, the prediction of stability over time gives substantial validity to the diagnosis.
- Relatives of bipolar probands with early age at onset have a greater risk than relatives of probands with late onset.

References

Andreasen NC, Rice JP, Endicott J, et al: The family history approach to diagnosis: how useful is it? Arch Gen Psychiatry 43:421–429, 1986

Cox N, Reich T, Rice JP, et al: Segregation and linkage analysis of bipolar and major depressive illnesses in multigenerational pedigrees. J Psychiatr Res 23:109–123, 1989

Endicott J, Spitzer RL: A diagnostic interview: the Schedule for Affective Disorders and Schizophrenia. Arch Gen Psychiatry 35:837–844, 1978

Fienberg SE, Mason W: Identification and estimation of age-period-cohort models in the analysis of discrete archival data, in Sociological Methodology. Edited by Schuessler KR. San Francisco, CA, Jossey-Bass, 1979, pp 1–67

Gershon ES, Hamovit S, Guroff JJ, et al: A family study of schizoaffective, bipolar I, bipolar II, unipolar, and normal control probands. Arch Gen Psychiatry 39:1157–1167, 1982

Klerman GL, Lavori PW, Rice JP, et al: Birth-cohort trends in rates of major depressive disorder among relatives of patients with affective disorder. Arch Gen Psychiatry 42:689–693, 1985

Kraemer HC: Ramifications of a population model for κ as a coefficient of reliability. Psychometrika 44:461–472, 1979

Lavori PW, Warshaw M, Klerman G, et al: Secular trends in lifetime onset of MDD stratified by selected sociodemographic risk factors. J Psychiatr Res 27:95–109, 1993

Major Depressive Disorder Working Group of the Psychiatric GWAS Consortium: A mega-analysis of genome-wide association studies for major depressive disorder. Mol Psychiatry April 3, 2012 [Epub ahead of print]

Psychiatric GWAS Consortium Bipolar Disorder Working Group: Large-scale genome-wide association analysis of bipolar disorder identifies a new susceptibility locus near *ODZ4*. Nat Genet 43:977–983, 2011

Rice JP, Todorov AA: Stability of diagnosis: application to phenotype definition. Schizophr Bull 20:185–190, 1994

Rice JP, Reich T, Andreasen NC, et al: Sex related differences in depression: familial evidence. J Affect Disord 71:199–210, 1984

Rice JP, McDonald-Scott P, Endicott J, et al: The stability of diagnosis with an application to bipolar II disorder. Psychiatry Res 19:285–296, 1986

Rice JP, Endicott J, Knesevich MA, et al: The estimation of diagnostic sensitivity using stability data: an application to major depressive disorder. J Psychiatr Res 21:337–345, 1987a

Rice JP, Reich T, Andreasen NC, et al: The familial transmission of bipolar illness. Arch Gen Psychiatry 44:441–447, 1987b

Rice JP, Rochberg N, Endicott J, et al: Stability of psychiatric diagnoses: an application to the affective disorders. Arch Gen Psychiatry 49:824–830, 1992

Rice JP, Neuman RJ, Saccone NL, et al: Age and birth cohort effects on rates of alcohol dependence. Alcohol Clin Exp Res 27:93–99, 2003

Robins E, Guze SB: Establishment of diagnostic validity in psychiatric illness: its application to schizophrenia. Am J Psychiatry 126:107–111, 1970

Robins LN, Helzer JE, Weissman MM, et al: Lifetime prevalence of specific psychiatric disorders in three sites. Arch Gen Psychiatry 41:949–958, 1984

Sklar P, Smoller JW, Fan J, et al: Whole-genome association study of bipolar disorder. Mol Psychiatry 13:558–569, 2008

Slater E, Cowie V: The Genetics of Mental Disorders. London, Oxford University Press, 1971

Sturt E, Kumakura N, Der G: How depressing life is—lifetime morbidity risk for depressive disorder in the general population. J Affect Disord 7:109–122, 1984

Chapter 12

Clinical Course and Outcome of Unipolar Major Depression

Martin B. Keller, M.D.
Robert Boland, M.D.
Andrew Leon, Ph.D.
David Solomon, M.D.
Jean Endicott, Ph.D.
Chunshan Li, M.A.

THE BEGINNING of the twentieth century brought new insight to our understanding of manic-depressive illness. Kraepelin's observations led him to separate mood disorders from schizophrenia because of differences in their symptom profiles and long-term clinical course. He found that the course of depression was generally characterized by relatively brief episodes and that an undefined subgroup of patients had recurrent episodes from which they recovered and resumed their previous state of wellness.

In this chapter, we concentrate on time to recovery from episodes of unipolar major depression, time to recurrence, and predictors thereof on the basis of 30 years of prospective follow-up. The chapter complements Chapter 3 ("Dimensional Symptomatic Structure of the Long-Term Course of Unipolar Major Depressive Disorder"), which deals with all levels of severity of depressive symptoms during long-term follow-up, including those below the threshold for major or minor depressive episodes.

155

Understanding the course of depression is crucial to recognizing and treating the disorder. This understanding helps clinicians and patients decide when to initiate treatment, how long to treat, and how to anticipate the needs of a depressed patient. Various studies have clarified the high morbidity associated with depression, which is comparable to or greater than that for other chronic medical conditions (Hays et al. 1995; Murray and Lopez 1996).

Following Kraepelin and prior to the publication of data from the Collaborative Depression Study (CDS), relatively little was published on the course of unipolar depression. However, by the 1970s, several longitudinal studies had examined the course of depression. In 1979, a critical review of this literature found varying rates of single and multiple depressive episodes because of differences in methodology and sample composition and a lack of a consistent definition of recurrence (Zis and Goodwin 1979). The proportion of individuals with single episodes ranged from 0% (in a study of 1,027 subjects; Angst 1980) to 58% (in a study of 319 patients; Lundquist 1945), whereas the proportion of those with multiple episodes ranged from 18% (in the same study of 319 patients) to 80% (in a study of 1,104 patients; Perris 1968). In 1981, CDS investigators Keller and Shapiro (1981) found only a few studies that reported comprehensive data or information on the course of depression (Cardoret et al. 1980; Morrison et al. 1973; Paykel and Dienelt 1971; Perris 1966; Schapira et al. 1972). These studies also challenged Kraepelin's impression that complete recovery from an episode was a defining characteristic of unipolar depression. They showed both a wide range of recovery rates among patients (from 31% to 90%) and a substantial proportion of patients who were considered recovered but who still had residual symptoms. Differences in methodology made it difficult to compare results between studies, however. For example, Morrison and colleagues (1973) used a sample of inpatients whose condition was diagnosed with explicit diagnostic criteria that specified a minimum of 1 month of depressed mood accompanied by four of seven symptoms without a previous nonaffective disorder or a history of mania. Another study (Cardoret et al. 1980) sampled family practice outpatients who did not present with depression as the primary complaint.

The CDS began in the mid-1970s by developing and field testing the Schedule for Affective Disorders and Schizophrenia (SADS; Endicott and Spitzer 1978) and the Research Diagnostic Criteria (RDC; Spitzer et al. 1978), both of which were direct progenitors of the American Psychiatric Association's current *Diagnostic and Statistical Manual of Mental Disorders*. The CDS brought a clear and consistent method of assessment to the study of all the affective disorders. The use of specific diagnostic criteria, criterion-based definitions of recovery and relapse or recurrence, and prospective longitudinal follow-up assessments separated by relatively short intervals between assessments provided continuity and precision in describing long-term course of illness. This was in contrast to earlier studies that used cross-sectional, retrospective, or extended intervals requiring considerable recall of symptoms in between. The intervals of either 6 or 12 months between interviews provided the opportunity to collect detailed data shown to be reliable and valid (Keller et al. 1987).

We review the published data obtained with these methods through the course of the first 15 years of the study, as well as recently analyzed data from the later 15 years of the study for a total of 30 years of follow-up. The sample sizes vary in different CDS articles because analyses were done and articles published at different follow-up durations and for different subgroups with unipolar depression.

Studies on the Course of Depression Other Than the Collaborative Depression Study

Prior to the CDS, a few prospective follow-up studies of patients with mood disorders were done, and others were contemporary to the CDS (Table 12–1). Of these, the study by Angst and Preisig (1995) most closely resembled the CDS. That study, centered in Zurich, Switzerland, followed up on more than 400 patients for 25 years. It was limited, however, by the large amount of time that elapsed between interviews (5 years), which restricted the focus largely to episode duration and frequency.

Several of the studies that were conducted around the same time as the CDS had varied results, some showing a more and others a less pernicious course than the CDS. The disparities were largely a result of differing methodologies, including different definitions of recovery and recurrence, lack of structured interviews at baseline, and reliance on retrospective recall, often for long intervals of time. The Groningen Primary Care Study (Ormel et al. 1993), conducted in the Netherlands, found that 93% of depressed patients had remitted from their index episode by 1 year. In France, Limosin et al. (2004) found a recovery rate of 65% by 6 months, and the World Health Organization study (Barkow et al. 2003) reported that 67% of patients recovered by 12 months. Perhaps most surprising was the Longitudinal Investigation of Depression Outcomes (LIDO) study (Simon et al. 2004), which found that only 35% of patients reported having had a complete remission by 1 year; this lower-than-expected remission rate was probably a result of the conservative definition of recovery, which required complete remission of all major depressive disorder (MDD) symptoms.

TABLE 12–1. Prospective studies on the course of major depression

Study	N	Diagnosis	Follow-up intervals after intake	Length of follow-up
Collaborative Depression Study (CDS) 1978–2009	955	Outpatients and inpatients: unipolar and bipolar	6 months for 5 years, then annually	30 years
Angst and Presig 1995	406	Inpatients: unipolar and bipolar	5 years	25 years
Brodaty et al. 2001; Maj et al. 2002	145	Inpatients: unipolar only	6 months; 2, 6, and 15 years	15 years
Lee and Murray 1988; Nystrom 1979	89	Inpatients: unipolar only	18 years	18 years
Surtees and Barkley 1994	80	Inpatients: unipolar only	12 years	12 years
Maj et al. 1992	72	Outpatients and inpatients: unipolar only	6 months	5 years
Ormel et al. 1993	1,271 (screened), 340 (stage 2)	Outpatients (primary care): depression, anxiety, mixed anxiety depression	1 year	3.5 years
Limosin et al. 2004	492	Outpatients (primary care): unipolar	6 months	6 months
World Health Organization study (Barkow et al. 2003)	1,174	Outpatients (primary care): unipolar	12 months	12 months

TABLE 12–1. Prospective studies on the course of major depression (continued)

Study	N	Diagnosis	Follow-up intervals after intake	Length of follow-up
Longitudinal Investigation of Depression Outcomes (Simon et al. 2004)	1,117	Outpatients (primary care): unipolar	12 months	12 months
Mattisson et al. 2007	344	Community sample: unipolar	10, 25, and 50 years, variable	Maximum 50 years
Coryell et al. 1994	216	Relatives, control subjects, and spouses of CDS probands: unipolar and bipolar	Once	6 years
Goldberg and Harrow 2004	133	Inpatients: unipolar and bipolar	2, 4, 5, 7.5, and 10 years	10 years
Duggan et al. 1990	89	Inpatients: unipolar	Once	18 years
Surtees and Barkley 1994	80	Inpatients: unipolar	Once	12 years
Weissman et al. 1999	73	Inpatient adolescents: unipolar	Once	10–15 years
Geller et al. 2001	72	Inpatient prepubertal children: unipolar	2–5 and 10 years	10 years
Eaton et al. 2008	71	Community sample: unipolar	11 and 12 years	23 years
Smith and North 1988	69	Inpatients: unipolar	Once	11 years
Kennedy et al. 2004	61	Inpatients: unipolar	Every 3 months for 15 months, then once	8–11 years

Description of the Collaborative Depression Study

The methodology of the CDS (Katz and Klerman 1979) is described in detail elsewhere in this volume (see Chapter 2, "Collaborative Depression Study Procedures and Study Design").

The CDS was an observational study in that treatment was observed but not controlled by the investigators. However, the type and dose of each somatic psychotropic treatment were systematically recorded. Somatic treatments for depression included antidepressants, lithium, and electroconvulsive therapy.

Results were collected and reported throughout the length of the study, and reports from the CDS described progressively longer periods of follow-up. At the 10-year point in the study, the decision was made to include only prospectively observed episodes in the analyses of recovery and recurrence. During the first 10 years of the study, 92% of the patients recovered from their first prospectively observed episode. The analysis done at the end of the study (30 years) was based on the subset of subjects who for the entire study had only unipolar MDD and were prospectively observed. More specifically, from the original sample of 431 unipolar subjects, some subjects eventually had a bipolar mania, hypomania, or a mixed episode or schizoaffective mood episode during prospective follow-up, leaving a sample of 338 subjects who had unipolar MDD for the duration of their follow-up. Because we planned to study only MDD episodes prospectively observed in their entirety in the new analyses, we removed those subjects who recovered from the intake depressive episode but did not have a subsequent relapse, leaving 214 subjects who had prospectively observed MDD episodes.

Results From the Collaborative Depression Study and Discussion

The CDS has greatly expanded our knowledge of the course and outcome of depression. It generated compelling evidence that episodes of depression were more chronic and recurrent than originally thought and that the intervals between episodes were more likely to have subsyndromal symptoms with impairment than they were to lack any depressive symptoms. The implications of the CDS have influenced the design of many randomized clinical treatment trials and have helped inform many of the clinical dilemmas that practitioners are likely to encounter—some of which are presented and discussed in this section. To illustrate the clinical value of these data for practitioners, the CDS findings on the course and outcome of episodes of depression are presented in a clinical case scenario model based on the patient's history of depression when seeking treatment, including

- The presence and duration of prior episodes
- Whether patients have had prospectively observed prior episodes at the time of seeking treatment
- The number of prospectively observed prior episodes
- Whether patients have been well for at least 8 consecutive weeks and are showing signs of recurrence
- Whether patients have been well for at least 1 year before seeking treatment
- Whether patients have had symptoms of dysthymia or minor depression since they last had a major depressive episode and recovered
- Whether patients have substantial social and occupational dysfunction

Scenario 1—A patient with or without a history of treated or untreated episodes of MDD presents to a new clinician for treatment of MDD.

In Scenario 1, the CDS is of great help for predicting the likely recovery from and course of the first episode for which the clinician is seeing the patient, even if he or she had seen other clinicians previously.

Some studies just prior to the CDS suggested that many patients have a more chronic course of depression than had been previously thought. For example, in a prospective follow-up of 96 patients with MDD, one study (Rounsaville et al. 1980) found that 12% of the subjects had not recovered after 16 months. Similarly, in the Zurich study, Angst and Preisig (1995) reported that after 27 years of follow-up, about 13% of the patients did not recover from the episode of MDD that was present at study intake.

In the CDS, early analyses reported that 61 of 86 (71%) patients with unipolar major depression recovered from the index episode within the first year (Keller and Shapiro 1981). At intake, 75% were inpatients and 25% were outpatients, the median age was 35.5, and the majority were female (56 females vs. 45 males). Of those patients who did not recover from MDD in the first year, most still had not recovered after a much longer time. Overall, the median duration from onset of the index episode to recovery was 30 weeks. For patients who did not recover, the median duration of onset of the index episode to the end of the 1-year follow-up period was 99 weeks (Keller and Shapiro 1981). Also, recovery typically was characterized by a gradual rather than a sudden decrease in symptoms. In addition, the probability that a patient who is depressed at the start of a year will recover during that year decreased over time: the longer an individual was ill, the lower his or her chance to recover in the next year. By 2 years, about 20% of the original sample still had not recovered; thus, two-thirds of those who remained depressed at 1 year were still in their index episode of depression at 2 years (Keller et al. 1984).

Note that these analyses were done in a clinical sample, but a similar analysis was done in the nonclinical group of relatives, spouses, and control subjects as a single 6-year follow-up evaluation. This indicated that the cumulative probability of recovery from MDD for this sample, identified based on having an ill relative and not on whether they had sought treatment, was very similar to that for the probands (Coryell et al. 1994).

Scenario 2—A patient who recovered from his last episode of MDD returns to the same clinician after a recurrence of MDD.

As noted earlier, the median duration from onset of the index episode to recovery was 30 weeks. However, a significant advantage of the CDS was the ability to observe multiple prospective episodes of a mood disorder, which clinicians frequently encountered when treating the same patient over a period of years. We observed that the first prospectively observed episode was shorter in duration than the index episode. Among the 214 subjects who had prospectively observed MDD within 5 years of follow-up, 672 prospectively observed depressive episodes occurred. The median length of time in the first prospective episode of MDD before recovery was 23 weeks (SE = 3.6).

Scenario 3—A patient presents to the clinician for a subsequent (second or more) prospectively observed episode, which occurs when the same clinician treats at least several episodes over years.

The CDS observed episodes of depression beyond the first prospectively observed episode. In the first 10 years of follow-up, 88% recovered from their second prospectively observed episode, 92% recovered from their third episode, and 88% recovered from their fourth prospectively observed episode. (At this point in the study, 235 subjects had had at least one recurrent mood episode and had no change in diagnosis. Of that sample, 91% of the subjects were followed up for at least 5 years, and 76% were followed up for 10 years.) Thus, the rates of recovery were similar for subsequent episodes.

In the analyses of 214 subjects with prospectively observed MDD episodes without hypomania, mania, or schizoaffective episodes, followed up for up to 30 years, the time to recovery was similar for the duration of sequential episodes; the median was 20 weeks for the second prospective episode ($N=137$; SE = 3.0), 20 weeks for the third ($N=91$; SE = 2.7), 25 weeks for the fourth ($N=72$; SE = 3.8), and 25 weeks ($N=51$; SE = 3.4) for the fifth prospectively observed episode.

Scenario 4—A patient presents in an episode of MDD that has lasted for 5 years or longer.

The 1992 analyses of the 5-year data set led to unanticipated results that had a major effect on redefining the field's knowledge of the clinical course of MDD (Keller et al. 1992). These described 431 subjects who entered into the CDS with a diagnosis of MDD who never had mania, hypomania, dysthymia, or schizoaffective disorder. Of these, 12% had not recovered from their index episode within 5 years. Those with more severe MDD symptoms were less likely to recover than those with a moderate level of symptoms. On the whole, the longer an individual was ill, the lower was that individual's chance to recover.

As noted, the 10-year follow-up analyses relied on data from the first prospectively observed episode of depression because these data did not require retrospective recall. By 10 years, 8% of the patients had not recovered from their first prospectively observed episode (Solomon et al. 1997); that number decreased to about 6% by 15 years (Keller and Boland 1998). It is noteworthy that the recovery rate in this prospectively observed sample was similar to earlier reports from the index episode: Mueller and colleagues (1996) reported that 10 years after the index episode, 93% of patients had recovered. For those who remained in a major depressive episode for the first 5 years of the study, 38% recovered within the next 5 years.

The data after 15 years were determined from the analysis of the 214 subjects at the end of the study who had had a prospectively observed episode of depression and continued to carry a diagnosis of unipolar MDD. In patients with episodes of depression lasting longer than 15 years, the rates of recovery were about 4% annually from year 15 through the 30 years of the study.

These results from the CDS challenged the earlier theories that sociodemographic variables such as age, gender, and marital status influence the course of MDD. Among the predictors associated with recovery, chronicity was most highly correlated with the cumulative time that the subject was depressed. In the first year of the study, contrary to the common belief at the time, married patients did not have a better rate of recovery. The analysis at 5-year follow-up suggested that anxiety symptoms were associated with more severe and persistent illness (Coryell et al. 1992b). By the 10-year analysis of the study, there were few predictors of recovery based on clinical variables at time of study enrollment. Many sociodemographic and clinical variables were studied, but none of these consistently influenced the time to recovery (Solomon et al. 1997), although at 20 years, psychosocial impairment predicted poor recovery (Solomon et al. 2008).

These data show that although most patients recover from an episode of depression, a substantial number of patients do not, and their likelihood of recovery declines the longer that they remain depressed.

Note that these findings were for clinical populations who were enrolled while seeking care at tertiary care centers and that these data might not be generalizable to patients who are not in tertiary care. Coryell and colleagues

(1991), however, described a large group of relatives of probands, control subjects, and spouses with two evaluations 6 years apart. Among those who recalled having had major depression before the initial interview, predictors of recurrence were young age, but not sex, number of symptoms recalled from their worst depressive episode, and the presence of minor depressive symptoms at the time of the initial evaluation. Risks for first onset during the interval included female sex, young age, and a history of nonaffective illness (Coryell et al. 1992a).

Scenario 5—After successful treatment of a first prospective MDD episode, a patient who has been well for more than 8 weeks is at high risk for subsequent recurrence of MDD.

Studies prior to the CDS suggested that MDD is a more recurrent illness than originally thought. These studies looked at recovery from the index episode and reported on the rate of occurrence of a second (first prospective) episode. One study (Weissman et al. 1976) found that among 150 women who recovered from MDD, two-thirds had a recurrence of depression during follow-up lasting for at least 1 year. Rao and Nammalvar (1977), examining more than 100 cases of depression in India with a follow-up of between 3 and 13 years, found that only about 25% of the original group reported no recurrence of symptoms. Angst (1992), in a 10-year follow-up of more than 1,000 patients, found that three-quarters of the sample had one or more recurrences of depression. Although Angst examined several sociodemographic variables, none significantly predicted the recurrence.

In the CDS, earlier analyses also suggested a high rate of recurrence. In the first year of follow-up, 74% of the 75 patients with unipolar depression recovered from the index episode, and 36% of those who recovered experienced another mood episode within the first year of follow-up (Keller and Shapiro 1981). After 2 years of follow-up, 40% of 97 subjects had a second episode of MDD (Keller et al. 1984). These rates of recurrence in the CDS group increased as the study progressed; the recurrence rate was 60% of the 431 total subjects eventually enrolled with MDD after 5 years (Keller et al. 1992), 65% of 319 subjects who recovered from their index episode (Solomon et al. 2000), and 85% of 380 subjects after 15 years (Mueller et al. 1999).

Depression secondary to other Axis I psychiatric disorders, older age at intake, and three or more prior episodes of MDD predicted recurrence within the first 2 years of follow-up (Keller et al. 1983b). After 5 years of follow-up, the most significant predictor of poor recovery was a high severity of symptoms (Keller et al. 1992).

At 10-year follow-up, the strongest predictor of recurrence was the number of previous episodes, with a 16% increased risk of recurrence with each subsequent episode (Solomon et al. 2000). After 15 years of follow-up, the predictors were female sex, longer episode prior to intake, greater number of prior episodes, and never marrying (Mueller et al. 1999).

More recent analyses on the 214 subjects who had no manic or hypomanic symptoms through the end of the study found that the rates of recurrence continued to increase, albeit more slowly, for the remainder of the study: 89% by 20 years and 91% by 25 and 30 years.

In analyzing predictors of recurrence for the 30-year data, several hypothesized predictors were tested with mixed-effects models that accounted for the correlation among multiple mood episodes within subjects. Although not predictive of recovery, comorbid anxiety and alcohol or substance abuse significantly predicted recurrence. The cumulative number of years depressed did not significantly predict recurrence.

The association between alcoholism and a poorer course of depression often has been reported and has been a consistent finding in the CDS. For example, in the CDS, Mueller et al. (1994) found that depressed subjects with alcoholism were half as likely as other patients to recover from their episode of MDD. In Chapter 8, "Comorbidity of Mood and Substance Use Disorders," Hasin and Kilcoyne provide a detailed review of substance abuse in the CDS.

Scenario 6—A patient with multiple past MDD episodes has been well for a meaningful period (e.g., 1 year) but is concerned about the risk of future depressive episodes.

As already noted, the long duration and prospective nature of the CDS provided an opportunity to prospectively observe the length of time until recurrence for patients with long periods of wellness between episodes. Data from the most recent analysis of the study indicated that the median time until recurrence was approximately 2 years (115 weeks).

When multiple well periods were analyzed, the length of the well period appeared to decrease with subsequent episodes. For the first well period (i.e., the period of wellness following recovery from the MDD episode at study intake), 50% continued to remain well at 3 years; for the second and third well periods, the median decreased to a little more than 2 years; and for the fourth and fifth well periods, it decreased to 91 and 94 weeks, respectively.

Thus, among these subjects, observed for up to 30 years, those who had at least one recurrence went on to have multiple recurrences. In addition, the duration of the well periods decreased with each subsequent episode for the first four episodes (substantially fewer subjects were available for the last observed episode).

This decrease in the duration of wellness is a relatively novel finding: previously, it was generally reported that the time to recurrence does not change over time. Earlier publications from the CDS did report that the length of time between MDD episodes progressively decreased with each episode (Solomon et al. 2000). However, for any single subject with multiple recurrences, the duration of wellness varied considerably. The data suggest that patients who have multiple recurrences of MDD are at risk for a worsening course of their disorder; these create a strong argument for preventive and early intervention treatment strategies.

Scenario 7—A patient whose MDD was successfully treated continues to have symptoms of dysthymia or minor depressive symptoms.

The concurrent presence of both dysthymia and major depression, or "double depression" (Keller and Shapiro 1982), was first reported in the literature by the CDS and is an important course modifier. By definition, patients with this disorder has a chronic course. The CDS found that many subjects, although recovering to the point that their symptoms no longer met the criteria for a major depressive episode, continued to have minor depressive symptoms sufficiently severe and chronic to justify a diagnosis of dysthymia. For example, at 5 years, of the 431 patients studied, 25 patients were still ill but below full criteria for major depression for most of the time (>130 weeks) (Keller et al. 1992).

Patients with double depression are also more likely to relapse into MDD. In the CDS, relapse was twice as likely for patients with double depression, compared with other depressed patients (Keller et al. 1983a).

Even when not reaching the level of a dysthymic disorder, the presence of any lingering depressive symptoms following an episode of MDD can have a deleterious effect on a patient's course. The CDS found that most patients who recover from MDD still have substantial subsyndromal symptoms and associated impairment in functioning. This degree of lingering impairment predicts subsequent relapse of MDD (Judd et al. 2000); these findings are also discussed in Chapter 3.

Scenario 8—A patient in an MDD episode experiences substantial social or occupational dysfunction.

Depression has a substantial, negative effect on a person's psychosocial functioning. Mild depressions, or even one symptom of depression, may result in psychosocial dysfunction (Judd et al. 2008). It thus appears that depressive symptoms in almost any amount are disabling, and as symptom level increases, so too does psychosocial impairment.

The CDS used the Range of Impaired Functioning Tool (LIFE-RIFT; Leon et al. 1999) to gather information on psychosocial functioning. The LIFE-RIFT was designed to measure psychosocial impairment and is a semistructured interview that targets functioning in four domains: life role function, interpersonal relationships, recreation, and global satisfaction. Each domain is rated on a five-point scale, with one representing no impairment and a high level of functioning and five indicating severe impairment.

In an early analysis of the psychosocial predictors of chronicity, Hirschfeld and colleagues (1986) found that the only psychosocial variable that predicted chronicity was increased neuroticism on self-reported inventories. However, the sample size was limited to 19 patients seen over 2 years.

In a review of the first 14 years of follow-up of 231 individuals with MDD, impairment in psychosocial functioning was associated with a decreased likelihood of recovery. As noted earlier, recovery was defined as 8 weeks with no symptoms or no more than one or two symptoms in a mild degree. When this definition of recovery was used, a 1 standard deviation increase in psychosocial impairment (about 3 LIFE-RIFT units) was associated with a 19% decrease in the probability of recovery. A more stringent definition of 8 weeks with no symptoms was also tested. An increase of 1 standard deviation in psychosocial impairment was associated with a 61% decrease in probability of recovery (Solomon et al. 1997).

Depression adversely affects psychosocial functioning. Analyses of functioning that incorporated all 30 years of prospective follow-up found that subjects who were currently in an episode of MDD had a LIFE-RIFT score that was approximately 4 points (>1 SD) higher than those who were currently in a well interval (mean=14.07; SD=3.03 vs. mean=10.24; SD=3.75). (The range of the LIFE-RIFT is 4 [no impairment] to 20 [severe impairment].) This is consistent with the finding reported in Chapter 3 of this volume that global ratings of psychosocial functioning increase or decrease significantly with each stepwise increase or decrease in level of depressive symptom severity within individual subjects over time. Thus, improvements in depressive symptoms are associated with improvements in functioning; this suggests that treatment may improve functioning and mood.

Somatic Treatment

A mean of 57% (SD=0.36) of patients were receiving some level of somatic treatment (defined as an antidepressant, lithium, or electroconvulsive therapy) while they were experiencing an episode of MDD. During well intervals, this percentage decreased to 37% (SD=0.38). The issue of the undertreatment of depression is discussed in detail in Chapter 14, "Undertreatment of Major Depression," and the issues of the effectiveness and safety of treatment are the subject of Chapter 9, "Treatment Effectiveness and Safety in the Longitudinal Course of Mood Disorders."

Future Directions

Future research must concentrate on four areas that the CDS was not able to sufficiently address: pathophysiology, genetics, the environment, and comorbidity.

1. **Pathophysiology**—We have yet to understand the underlying pathophysiology of depressive illness and have no means of evaluating this state directly. Several biological markers for mood have been reported, including rapid eye movement sleep dysfunction, dysfunction of the hypothalamic-pituitary-adrenal axis, and similar endocrine disturbances; however, no biological abnormalities have the specificity needed for a clinical test. Increased knowledge of the neurobiology of mood will allow more precise assessments and diagnoses at the onset of treatment and measurement of response to treatment.

2. **Genetics**—Similarly, we continue to search for genetic markers of a risk for depression. It has long been known that depressed patients, particularly patients with recurrent depression, have family histories strongly suggestive of a genetic inheritance of risk. Most promising have been reports of associations between early life stress, depression, and genes associated with the serotonin transporter. However, to date, no genetic association has been found consistently enough to be of clinical use in unipolar disorder. We hope that newer genetic techniques that allow rapid genotyping will begin to untangle the complex relation between genetic dispositions and mood disorders. See Chapter 11, "Family History and Genetic Studies in Mood Disorders," for a detailed discussion of the genetics of depression.

3. **Environment**—The role of the environment in depression, particularly the importance of adverse life events and their effect on depression, is another important area of study. As discussed, some current controversy exists regarding the role that stress plays in the etiology and maintenance of depression, and more work needs to be done to clarify these relations.

4. **Comorbidity**—The problems of comorbidity and its effect on the course of depression are important areas in need of investigation. Although literature in this area is growing, more work must be done to clarify the nature of the interaction between depression, comorbid nonaffective psychiatric disease, and comorbid medical disease.

Clinical Implications

- Before the Collaborative Depression Study, mood disorders most often were thought to be acute, single-episode diseases that were likely to show complete recovery when properly treated. Empirical evidence from the CDS has caused a paradigm shift in the understanding of mood disorders because moderate to severe mood disorders are often chronic illnesses that are likely to recur.
- Many individuals have residual subsyndromal symptoms and disabling psychosocial impairment when recovered from major episodes of depression for at least 2 months.
- A significant portion of individuals with major depression experienced a highly recurrent and chronic course of symptoms. Findings of the CDS suggested that randomized clinical trials should extend the length of study to better learn how long treatment must be maintained to significantly reduce the risk of recurrence. The CDS data on clinical course of major depressive disorder, including predictors, had a major influence on the specific design of the early long-term maintenance studies of recurrent MDD (Kupfer et al. 1992).
- Depression is a lifelong illness for a high proportion of affected individuals. However, for individual patients, we still cannot adequately predict who will develop only a single episode, who will go on to experience recurrent episodes with interepisode recovery, and who will become chronically depressed. Consequently, many patients are fated to endure the morbidity of major depressive episodes because of premature treatment withdrawal and inadequate treatment. We need to better target which patients should have long-term treatment and then determine which treatments will best prevent future episodes.
- Predictors of course that were significant early in the disease have weakened over time, suggesting a change in the nature of the illness, our inability to detect existing predictors, and the heterogeneous nature of the illness.
- Lack of patient adherence is a potential barrier to treatment efficacy; yet most of the studies discussed in this chapter did not collect such data. The CDS collected data on dose and duration of treatment. It did not, however, ascertain the physician's recommended treatment. Therefore, we do not know how well the medication use and physician recommendation agreed.

- Data are needed on adherence, including variables that may explain problems with adherence. To understand how adherence affects the long-term course of depression, we need to incorporate these data into long-term intervention and observational studies.
- Little information is available on the decision-making processes of physicians, which suggests that more than mere education will be needed to improve the process of initiating and maintaining treatment in patients with depression (see Chapter 14, "Undertreatment of Major Depression").

References

Angst J: [Course of unipolar depressive, bipolar manic-depressive, and schizoaffective disorders: results of a prospective longitudinal study.] (author's transl) (in German). Fortschr Neurol Psychiatr Grenzgeb 48:3–30, 1980

Angst J: Epidemiology of depression. Psychopharmacology (Berl) 106(suppl):S71–74, 1992

Angst J, Preisig M: Course of a clinical cohort of unipolar, bipolar and schizoaffective patients: results of a prospective study from 1959 to 1985. Schweiz Arch Neurol Psychiatr 146:5–16, 1995

Barkow K, Maier W, Ustun TB, et al: Risk factors for depression at 12-month follow-up in adult primary health care patients with major depression: an international prospective study. J Affect Disord 76:157–169, 2003

Brodaty H, Luscombe G, Peisak C, et al: A 25-year longitudinal, comparison study of the outcome of depression. Psychol Med 31:1347–1359, 2001

Cardoret R, Widner RB, Widner RB: Depression in family practice: long-term prognosis and somatic complaints. J Fam Pract 10:625–629, 1980

Coryell W, Endicott J, Keller MB: Predictors of relapse into major depressive disorder in a nonclinical population. Am J Psychiatry 148:1353–1358, 1991

Coryell W, Endicott J, Keller MB: Major depression in a nonclinical sample: demographic and clinical risk factors for first onset. Arch Gen Psychiatry 49:117–125, 1992a

Coryell W, Endicott J, Winokur G: Anxiety syndromes as epiphenomena of primary major depression: outcome and familial psychopathology. Am J Psychiatry 149:100–107, 1992b

Coryell W, Akiskal HS, Leon AC, et al: The time course of nonchronic major depressive disorder: uniformity across episodes and samples. National Institute of Mental Health Collaborative Program on the Psychobiology of Depression—Clinical Studies. Arch Gen Psychiatry 51:405–410, 1994

Duggan CF, Lee AS, Murray RM: Does personality predict long-term outcome in depression? Br J Psychiatry 157:19–24, 1990

Eaton WW, Shao H, Nestadt G, et al: Population based study of first onset and chronicity in major depressive disorder. Arch Gen Psychiatry 65:515–520, 2008

Endicott J, Spitzer RL: A diagnostic interview: the Schedule for Affective Disorders and Schizophrenia. Arch Gen Psychiatry 35:837–844, 1978

Geller B, Zimmerman B, Williams M, et al: Bipolar disorder at prospective follow-up of adults who had prepubertal major depressive disorder. Am J Psychiatry 158:125–127, 2001

Goldberg JF, Harrow M: Consistency of remission and outcome of bipolar and unipolar mood disorders: a 10-year prospective follow-up. J Affect Disord 81:123–131, 2004

Hays RD, Wells KB, Sherbourne CD, et al: Functioning and well-being outcomes of patients with depression compared with chronic general medical illnesses. Arch Gen Psychiatry 52:11–19, 1995

Hirschfeld RM, Klerman GL, Andreasen NC, et al: Psycho-social predictors of chronicity in depressed patients. Br J Psychiatry 148:648–654, 1986

Judd LL, Paulus MJ, Schettler PJ, et al: Does incomplete recovery from first lifetime major depressive episode herald a chronic course of illness? Am J Psychiatry 157:1501–1504, 2000

Judd LL, Schettler PJ, Solomon DA, et al: Psychosocial disability and work role function compared across the long-term course of bipolar I, bipolar II and unipolar major depressive disorders. J Affect Disord 108:49–58, 2008

Katz MM, Klerman GL: Introduction: overview of the clinical studies program. Am J Psychiatry 136:49–51, 1979

Keller MB, Boland RJ: Implications of failing to achieve successful long-term maintenance treatment of recurrent unipolar major depression. Biol Psychiatry 44:348–360, 1998

Keller MB, Shapiro RW: Major depressive disorder: initial results from a one-year prospective naturalistic follow-up study. J Nerv Ment Dis 169:761–768, 1981

Keller MB, Shapiro RW: Double depression: superimposition of acute depressive episodes on chronic depressive disorders. Am J Psychiatry 139:438–442, 1982

Keller MB, Lavori PW, Endicott J, et al: Double depression: two-year follow-up. Am J Psychiatry 140:689–694, 1983a

Keller MB, Lavori PW, Lewis CE, et al. Predictors of relapse in major depressive disorder. JAMA 250:3299–3304, 1983b

Keller MB, Klerman GL, Lavori PW, et al: Long-term outcome of episodes of major depression: clinical and public health significance. JAMA 252:788–792, 1984

Keller MB, Lavori PW, Friedman B, et al: The Longitudinal Interval Follow-up Evaluation: a comprehensive method for assessing outcome in prospective longitudinal studies. Arch Gen Psychiatry 44:540–548, 1987

Keller MB, Lavori PW, Mueller TI, et al: Time to recovery, chronicity, and levels of psychopathology in major depression: a 5-year prospective follow-up of 431 subjects. Arch Gen Psychiatry 49:809–816, 1992

Kennedy N, Abbott R, Paykel ES: Longitudinal syndromal and sub-syndromal symptoms after severe depression: 10-year follow-up study. Br J Psychiatry 184:330–336, 2004

Kupfer DJ, Frank E, Perel JM, et al: Five-year outcome for maintenance therapies in recurrent depression. Arch Gen Psychiatry 49:769–773, 1992

Lee AS, Murray RM: The long-term outcome of Maudsley depressives. Br J Psychiatry 153:741–751, 1988

Leon AC, Solomon DA, Mueller TI, et al: The range of impaired functioning tool (LIFE-RIFT): a brief measure of functional impairment. Psychol Med 29:869–878, 1999

Limosin F, Loze JY, Zylberman-Bouhassira M, et al: The course of depressive illness in general practice. Can J Psychiatry 49:119–123, 2004

Lundquist G: Prognosis in manic-depressive psychoses. Acta Psychiatr Scand 20 (suppl 35):5–96, 1945

Maj M, Veltro F, Pirozzi R, et al: Pattern of recurrence of illness after recovery from an episode of major depression: a prospective study. Am J Psychiatry 149:795–800, 1992

Maj M, Pirozzi R, Magliano L, et al: The prognostic significance of "switching" in patients with bipolar disorder: a 10-year prospective follow-up study. Am J Psychiatry 159:1711–1717, 2002

Mattisson C, Bogren M, Horstmann V, et al: The long-term course of depressive disorders in the Lundby Study. Psychol Med 37:883–891, 2007

Morrison J, Winokur G, Crowe R, et al: The Iowa 500: the first follow-up. Arch Gen Psychiatry 29:678–682, 1973

Mueller TI, Lavori PW, Keller MB, et al: Prognostic effect of the variable course of alcoholism on the 10-year course of depression. Am J Psychiatry 151:701–706, 1994

Mueller TI, Keller MB, Leon AC, et al: Recovery after 5 years of unremitting major depressive disorder. Arch Gen Psychiatry 53:794–799, 1996

Mueller TI, Leon AC, Keller MB, et al: Recurrence after recovery from major depressive disorder during 15 years of observational follow-up. Am J Psychiatry 156:1000–1006, 1999

Murray CJ, Lopez AD: Evidence-based health policy—lessons from the Global Burden of Disease Study. Science 274(5288):740–743, 1996

Nystrom S: Depression: factors related to 10-year prognosis. Acta Psychiatr Scand 60:225–238, 1979

Ormel J, Oldehinkel T, Brilman E, et al: Outcome of depression and anxiety in primary care: a three-wave 3 1/2-year study of psychopathology and disability. Arch Gen Psychiatry 50:759–766, 1993

Paykel ES, Dienelt MN: Suicide attempts following acute depression. J Nerv Ment Dis 153:234–243, 1971

Perris C: A study of bipolar (manic-depressive) and unipolar recurrent depressive psychoses: introduction. Acta Psychiatr Scand Suppl 194: 9–14, 1966

Perris C: The course of depressive psychoses. Acta Psychiatr Scand 44:238–248, 1968

Rao AV, Nammalvar N: The course and outcome in depressive illness: a follow-up study of 122 cases in Madurai, India. Br J Psychiatry 130:392–396, 1977

Rounsaville BJ, Prusoff BA, Padian N: The course of nonbipolar, primary major depression: a prospective 16-month study of ambulatory patients. J Nerv Ment Dis 168:406–411, 1980

Schapira K, Roth M, Kerr TA, et al: The prognosis of affective disorders: the differentiation of anxiety states from depressive illnesses. Br J Psychiatry 121:175–181, 1972

Simon GE, Fleck M, Lucas R, et al: Prevalence and predictors of depression treatment in an international primary care study. Am J Psychiatry 161:1626–1634, 2004

Smith EM, North CS: Familial subtypes of depression: a longitudinal perspective. J Affect Disord 14:145–154, 1988

Solomon DA, Keller MB, Leon AC, et al: Recovery from major depression: a 10-year prospective follow-up across multiple episodes. Arch Gen Psychiatry 54:1001–1006, 1997

Solomon DA, Keller MB, Leon AC, et al: Multiple recurrences of major depressive disorder. Am J Psychiatry 157:229–233, 2000

Solomon DA, Leon AC, Coryell W, et al: Predicting recovery from episodes of major depression. J Affect Disord 107:285–291, 2008

Spitzer RL, Endicott J, Robins E: Research Diagnostic Criteria: rationale and reliability. Arch Gen Psychiatry 35:773–782, 1978

Surtees PG, Barkley C: Future imperfect: the long-term outcome of depression. Br J Psychiatry 164:327–341, 1994

Weissman MM, Kasl SV, Kerman GL: Follow-up of depressed women after maintenance treatment. Am J Psychiatry 133:757–760, 1976

Weissman MM, Wolk S, Goldstein RB, et al: Depressed adolescents grown up. JAMA 281:1707–1713, 1999

Zis AP, Goodwin FK: Major affective disorder as a recurrent illness: a critical review. Arch Gen Psychiatry 36 (8 Spec No):835–839, 1979

CHAPTER 13

Predictors of Course and Outcome of Bipolar Disorder

William H. Coryell, M.D.

PATIENTS WITH BIPOLAR disorder, their family members, and their clinicians need to know how long the illness is likely to last, whether and when it might recur, how it might evolve over time, and in what ways it might affect their lives. Answers to these questions derive from studies that describe the course of bipolar illness in general but more particularly from those that consider the prognostic importance of features that vary across individuals with bipolar disorder. These features include demographics, symptom quality, phase of illness, early course of illness, personality, past response to treatment, and family history.

The Collaborative Depression Study (CDS) is uniquely suited to describe prognosis in bipolar disorder because of its sample size, length of follow-up, and the thoroughness of both baseline and follow-up standardized assessments. As have many other studies, the CDS has described times to, and predictors of, remission from index episodes and first recurrences. CDS data have gone further, however, and have spoken to the timing of recurrences over lengthy periods, long-term illness burden, and the possible evolution of the illness over decades as reflected in changes in cycle length and symptom persistence.

Other chapters have included bipolar disorder data in their discussions of psychotic features, alcohol abuse, treatment effectiveness, and diagnostic stability. In particular, in Chapter 7, "Development of Mania or Hypomania in the Course of Unipolar Major Depression," Fiedorowicz et al. focus on changes in polarity, and in Chapter 4, "Dimensional Symptomatic Structure of the Long-Term Course of Bipolar I and Bipolar II Disorders," Judd et al. focus on the time spent in specific categories of illness polarity and severity, rates of changes in polarity, the psychosocial effect of different severity levels of depressive and manic spectrum symptoms, and the considerable importance of residual symptoms during periods of recovery. Here I emphasize how demographics, phenomenology, early illness course, and family history are related to the course of bipolar illness.

Methods

In Chapter 2 ("Collaborative Depression Study Procedures and Study Design"), Endicott describes CDS methods generally, but certain aspects should be emphasized here. Research Diagnostic Criteria (RDC) for a manic episode are essentially identical to those provided in DSM-IV-TR (American Psychiatric Association 2000), but the RDC did not discount episodes that follow somatic treatment and did not exclude symptoms possibly caused by the effects of a substance or medical illness. The RDC for hypomanic episode require two of the seven listed symptoms, or three if the mood is only irritable, whereas DSM-IV-TR requires three symptoms, or four if the mood is only irritable.

The RDC definition of schizoaffective disorder was much broader than that of DSM-IV-TR and required only the presence of one Schneiderian first-rank symptom (e.g., delusions and thought broadcasting) (Rosen et al. 2011) in the company of an otherwise manic syndrome. Many patients with an RDC diagnosis of schizoaffective disorder therefore would receive a diagnosis of manic disorder with mood-incongruent psychotic features in DSM-IV-TR. Some of the CDS analyses on bipolar illness excluded patients with diagnoses of schizoaffective mania, whereas others excluded only those with the mainly schizophrenic subtype, a category that overlaps considerably with DSM-IV-TR schizoaffective disorder.

Table 13–1 briefly describes the CDS sample of bipolar patients. Note that many who ended the study with a diagnosis of bipolar I or II disorder began with a nonbipolar diagnosis. Some CDS analyses confined their diagnostic groupings to those with an intake diagnosis of bipolar disorder, whereas others characterized as having bipolar illness anyone who had hypomanic or manic episodes during follow-up despite having had no such history prior to the study entry.

Outcomes

Episode Duration

Reports from the CDS concerning episode length began with descriptions of the episodes present at study intake (Coryell et al. 1989; Keller 1988; Keller et

TABLE 13–1. Collaborative Depression Study bipolar patients with at least 1 year of follow-up

	Bipolar II	Bipolar I
N	144	282
Sex,% female	66.0	53.9
Age, mean (SD)	35.9 (13.4)	36.5 (13.1)
Baseline diagnosis, n (%)		
Unipolar	62	40
Bipolar II	80	15
Bipolar I	—	216
Inpatient at intake (%)	66.0	90.4

al. 1986, 1992), moved to descriptions of prospectively observed episodes (Coryell et al. 1989, 2001; Fiedorowicz et al. 2012; Keller et al. 1993; Turvey et al. 1999a), and finally presented data that pooled multiple prospectively observed episodes (Mysels et al. 2007; Solomon et al. 2009, 2010).

The first of these reports found that mixed or cycling episodes had the longest time to recovery followed by pure depressive episodes and then by pure manic episodes (Keller 1988; Keller et al. 1986). The corresponding proportions that remained ill after 1 year of follow-up were 32%, 22%, and 7%. Later, with data from 5 years of follow-up, we showed that time to recovery for bipolar I, bipolar II, and nonbipolar groups overlapped closely and that recovery accumulated most rapidly in the first year and much less rapidly in the second year and beyond (Coryell et al. 1989). The likelihood of near-term recovery increased as weekly severity ratings decreased, indicating that most recoveries develop gradually (Keller et al. 1992).

One analysis that used prospectively observed episodes addressed the question of whether lithium discontinuation was followed by a poor lithium response in a subsequent episode (Coryell et al. 1998). It was not; new manic syndromes resolved somewhat more rapidly after the resumption of lithium than they had when lithium was administered in the index episode. This is also discussed in Chapter 9, "Treatment Effectiveness and Safety in the Longitudinal Course of Mood Disorders."

Subsequent work asked whether the polarity of onset of bipolar I disorder showed stability across multiple episodes and whether the onset phase type was consistently associated with time to episode recovery (Turvey et al. 1999b). Some stability was, in fact, apparent because those whose index episode began with a manic phase were much more likely to begin their first, second, and third prospectively observed episodes with mania than were those whose index episode began with depression. Moreover, episodes beginning with depressive phases were longer than those beginning with manic phases in each of the first three prospectively observed episodes. Other analyses showed that the longer times to recovery associated with an index mixed or cycling episode also occurred in the first prospectively observed episode (Keller et al. 1993).

The further lengthening of follow-up duration correspondingly increased the number of prospectively observed episodes available for analysis such that 219 patients with bipolar I disorder had at least one prospectively observed episode and 102 had at least five (Solomon et al. 2009, 2010), for a total of 1,208 episodes available for analysis. Among episodes without cycling, the median duration of major depressive episodes was 15 weeks, which was twice that for manic episodes (7 weeks) and minor depressive episodes (7 weeks) and five times longer than that for hypomanic episodes (3 weeks). Episodes with cycling that involved either or both major depression and mania had much longer median times to recovery (42 weeks), particularly if they included mixed (combined polarity) phases (61 weeks). With episode type present in a mixed-effect grouped-time survival analysis model, significant predictors of longer time to recovery were high severity at the episode's onset and higher amounts of prospectively observed cumulative morbidity expressed as symptom persistence.

Recurrence

As have nearly all other comparisons of nonbipolar and bipolar groups, the CDS has consistently shown relapse rates to be substantially higher among bipolar patients than among unipolar patients (Coryell et al. 1987, 1989; Winokur et al. 1993a). For both unipolar and bipolar depressions, the time elapsed from the most recent episode was strongly associated with near-term risk for recurrence (Coryell et al. 1995). The likelihood of recurrence in the ensuing 6 months for bipolar I disorder has been shown to range from 36% when the preceding episode has ended 4–12 months previously, to 18% if 1–2 years has passed, and to 10% if at least 3 years have past. Eventually, the likelihood of relapse was high even for those who had at one point been in remission for at least 3 years. At 7 years, 82% had experienced a new episode of mania or major depression. High rates of recurrence were seen as well for patients taking lithium prophylaxis, even though compliance, as evidenced by therapeutic lithium levels, was apparently good.

The nature of the preceding episode also exerted an influence on near-term risk for relapse such that previous mixed or cycling episodes portended higher likelihoods (Keller et al. 1993). A family history of mania also increased risks for relapse in the first 5 years to a modest but significant degree (Winokur et al. 1993b). Interestingly, as described in Chapter 7 of this volume, the link between a bipolar family and risk for recurrence reemerged in a very recent analysis of patients who entered the CDS with a diagnosis of unipolar disorder but who eventually developed an episode of mania or hypomania (Fiedorowicz et al. 2012). In a multivariate model with age at onset, the presence of an antidepressant at the time of first switching, and the presence of psychotic features, only a family history of bipolar disorder significantly predicted a shorter time to a new episode of hypomania or mania.

One CDS finding made possible by the length of follow-up and the frequency of assessment bears on the validity of the "kindling hypothesis" (Post et al. 1986). This hypothesis holds that repeated bipolar episodes sensitize an individual to more readily develop subsequent episodes and is based largely on the observation that the time from the start of one episode to the next appears to shorten as the lifetime number of episodes increases. Evidence for this, however, derives almost entirely from retrospective studies (Roy-Byrne et al. 1985), an approach open to the artifact of a poorer recall of those episodes that occurred in the more remote past. By contrast, prospective CDS data have consistently shown no trends toward decreasing times to recurrence across multiple, prospectively observed bipolar disorder episodes (Turvey et al. 1999b; Winokur et al. 1994).

Twenty-seven patients began follow-up in a manic episode and had no history of depressive episodes (Solomon et al. 2003). The observation that in only 7 patients did depressive episodes fail to develop during a follow-up of 15–20 years indicates that a small proportion of bipolar I patients appear to have true unipolar mania.

Symptom Burden

Many efforts to describe the course of bipolar disorder have used the timing of episode resolution and recurrence as the sole symptom-based measure. Although useful, this approach fails to capture the overall proportion of time in episodes and the severity of symptoms over extended periods. Such measures were proposed by Abou-Saleh and Coppen (1986) and have been variably termed as *affective morbidity* or *symptom burden*. They have been of particular value in the quantification of symptoms over a long period, and the CDS has increasingly used them as the follow-up period has grown.

One use was to define a poor outcome group in the fifteenth year of follow-up as those patients with bipolar I disorder who were in episodes of major depression or mania throughout that year (Coryell et al. 1998). A regression analysis determined that only poor optimal functioning in the 5 years preceding study intake and the persistence of depressive symptoms in the first 2 years of follow-up distinguished the poor outcome group from the remaining patients.

A symptom persistence measure was then used to examine whether family history of bipolar illness is associated with the quality of lithium response as reflected in symptom levels during lithium therapy (Coryell et al. 2000). Contrary to prior research (Grof et al. 1994, 2002), family history had no bearing on morbidity levels during lithium therapy. Instead, a family history positive for major depressive disorder without bipolar disorder was associated with higher symptom levels.

Psychotic features within the index episode were shown to be predictive not of time to remission or recurrence but of time in a depressive or manic episode during 15 years of observation (Coryell et al. 2001), much as psychotic features were associated with increased symptom burden in unipolar depression (see Chapter 6, "Psychotic Features in Major Depressive and Manic Episodes"). Bipolar and unipolar groups did not differ in the relation of baseline psychotic features to the number of weeks with active psychosis during follow-up. However, the presence of psychotic features in baseline depressive episodes was strongly predictive of the subsequent number of weeks with active psychosis. The presence of psychotic features during index manic episodes, in contrast, was not associated with the later persistence of psychosis.

We also used time in mood disorder episodes to describe the prognostic effects of rapid-cycling bipolar disorder (Coryell et al. 2003). Although four of five prospectively identified cases of rapid cycling ceased this pattern during the ensuing 2 years, rapid cycling was associated with persistently greater likelihoods of depressive symptoms for the remainder of follow-up.

The CDS assessed a variety of course variables measured in the first 5 years of follow-up as predictive of affective burden index in the second 5 years (Mysels et al. 2007). This measure took into account both time in mood disorder episodes and the intensity of the symptoms during episodes. Although the variables tested for their prognostic weight included frequency and character of switches between mania and depression, number of episodes, and weeks of drug or alcohol abuse, a multivariate analysis identified only the weeks of mania, hypomania, or mixed states in the first 5 years and, more strongly, the number of weeks in minor or major depressive episodes as predictive of the affective burden index in the second 5 years. With these data in the model, other variables were no longer significantly predictive, although many had correlated with later affective morbidity when tested in univariate analyses.

The size and duration of the CDS allowed us to ask whether symptom persistence in bipolar I disorder changed with increasing age and whether any such changes differed across youngest, middle, and oldest age groups (Coryell et al. 2009). Analyses found significantly increased depressive morbidity, but not manic or hypomanic morbidity, across four 5-year epochs for the youngest (18–29 years) and middle (30–44 years) age groups but not in patients who were older than 44 years at the study's beginning.

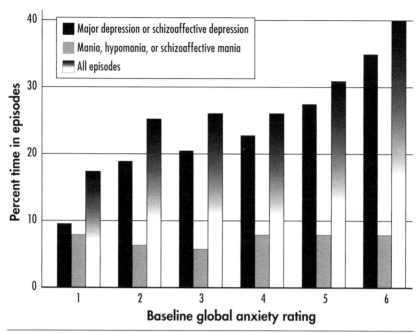

FIGURE 13–1. Baseline global anxiety rating and subsequent percentage of time in depressive or manic episodes in 427 patients with bipolar disorder.

Most recently, we have considered the long-term prognostic importance of baseline anxiety symptoms on subsequent course (Coryell et al. 2009). Two six-point ratings from the baseline diagnostic interview, one for somatic anxiety (e.g., physiological concomitants of anxiety) and the other for psychic anxiety as measured by the patient's subjective rating of anxiety intensity, quantified the intensity of the anxiety reported by patients. The sum of these two items showed a strong stepwise relation to the proportion of weeks in depressive episodes throughout 2 decades of follow-up, with little diminution of these effects across several decades. Notably, comorbid anxiety disorders were not predictive of depressive morbidity.

The importance of a summed intensity of six individual anxiety symptoms for subsequent depressive morbidity was similarly tested (Coryell et al. 2012). A stepwise relation between the intensity of baseline anxiety symptoms and subsequent morbidity again emerged for both bipolar and unipolar patients (Figure 13–1). The relations still held for the 5 years assessed between 20 and 25 years. This outcome indicates that a high level of anxiety during a depressive episode denotes a type of illness that features persistent depressive morbidity rather than characterizing only a particular type of episode.

Clinical Implications

- Mood episodes that include cycling, particularly those beginning with a depressive phase, last longer than those that do not.
- The time elapsed from the last episode predicts the short-term risk for recurrence, as does the presence of cycling in the previous episode.
- The persistence of depressive symptoms predicts higher morbidity in the long term.
- Psychotic features within manic episodes are associated with an increased long-term symptom burden but not with a higher likelihood of persistent psychosis.
- The time to episode recurrence does not shorten with repeated episodes.
- Rapid cycling eventually ceases in the large majority of cases but portends greater long-term symptom burden.
- High severity of anxiety symptoms during a bipolar depressive episode denotes a type of bipolar illness with substantially more long-term depressive morbidity.

References

Abou-Saleh MT, Coppen A: Who responds to prophylactic lithium? J Affect Disord 10:115–125, 1986

American Psychiatric Association: Diagnostic and Statistical Manual of Mental Disorders, 4th Edition, Text Revision. Washington, DC, American Psychiatric Association, 2000

Coryell W, Andreasen NC, Endicott J, et al: The significance of past mania or hypomania in the course and outcome of major depression. Am J Psychiatry 144:309–315, 1987

Coryell W, Keller M, Endicott J, et al: Bipolar II illness: course and outcome over a five-year period. Psychol Med 19:129–141, 1989

Coryell W, Endicott J, Maser JD, et al: The likelihood of recurrence in bipolar affective disorder: the importance of episode recency. J Affect Disord 33:201–206, 1995

Coryell W, Solomon D, Leon AC, et al: Lithium discontinuation and subsequent effectiveness. Am J Psychiatry 155:895–898, 1998

Coryell W, Akiskal H, Leon AC, et al: Family history and symptom levels during treatment for bipolar I affective disorder. Biol Psychiatry 47:1034–1042, 2000

Coryell W, Leon AC, Turvey C, et al: The significance of psychotic features in manic episodes: a report from the NIMH collaborative study. J Affect Disord 67:79–88, 2001

Coryell W, Solomon D, Turvey C, et al: The long-term course of rapid-cycling bipolar disorder. Arch Gen Psychiatry 60:914–920, 2003

Coryell W, Solomon DA, Fiedorowicz JG, et al: Anxiety and outcome in bipolar disorder. Am J Psychiatry 166:1238–1243, 2009

Coryell W, Solomon D, Leon A, et al: A dissection of the effects of anxiety features on the long-term course of depressive disorders. Br J Psychiatry 200:210–215, 2012

Fiedorowicz JG, Endicott J, Solomon DA, et al: Course of illness following prospectively observed mania or hypomania in individuals presenting with unipolar depression. Bipolar Disord 14:664–671, 2012

Grof P, Alda M, Grof E, et al: Lithium response and genetics of affective disorders. J Affect Disord 32:85–95, 1994

Grof P, Duffy A, Carazzoni P, et al: Is response to prophylactic lithium a familial trait? J Clin Psychiatry 63:942–947, 2002

Keller MB: The course of manic-depressive illness. J Clin Psychiatry 49(suppl):4–7, 1988

Keller MB, Lavori PW, Coryell W, et al: Differential outcome of pure manic, mixed/cycling, and pure depressive episodes in patients with bipolar illness. JAMA 255:3138–3142, 1986

Keller MB, Lavori PW, Mueller TI, et al: Time to recovery, chronicity, and levels of psychopathology in major depression: a 5-year prospective follow-up of 431 subjects. Arch Gen Psychiatry 49:809–816, 1992

Keller MB, Lavori PW, Coryell W, et al: Bipolar I: a five-year prospective follow-up. J Nerv Ment Dis 181:238–245, 1993

Mysels DJ, Endicott J, Nee J, et al: The association between course of illness and subsequent morbidity in bipolar I disorder. J Psychiatr Res 41:80–89, 2007

Post RM, Rubinow DR, Ballenger JC: Conditioning and sensitisation in the longitudinal course of affective illness. Br J Psychiatry 149:191–201, 1986

Rosen C, Grossman LS, Harrow M, et al: Diagnostic and prognostic significance of Schneiderian first-rank symptoms: a 20-year longitudinal study of schizophrenia. Compr Psychiatry 52:126–131, 2011

Roy-Byrne P, Post RM, Uhde TW, et al: The longitudinal course of recurrent affective illness: life chart data from research patients at the NIMH. Acta Psychiatr Scand Suppl 317:1–34, 1985

Solomon DA, Leon AC, Endicott J, et al: Unipolar mania over the course of a 20-year follow-up study. Am J Psychiatry 160:2049–2051, 2003

Solomon DA, Leon AC, Endicott J, et al: Empirical typology of bipolar I mood episodes. Br J Psychiatry 195:525–530, 2009

Solomon DA, Leon AC, Coryell WH, et al: Longitudinal course of bipolar I disorder: duration of mood episodes. Arch Gen Psychiatry 67:339–347, 2010

Turvey CL, Coryell WH, Arndt S, et al: Polarity sequence, depression, and chronicity in bipolar I disorder. J Nerv Ment Dis 187:181–187, 1999a

Turvey CL, Coryell WH, Solomon DA, et al: Long-term prognosis of bipolar I disorder. Acta Psychiatr Scand 99:110–119, 1999b

Winokur G, Coryell W, Endicott J, et al: Further distinctions between manic-depressive illness (bipolar disorder) and primary depressive disorder (unipolar depression). Am J Psychiatry 150:1176–1181, 1993a

Winokur G, Coryell W, Keller M, et al: A prospective follow-up of patients with bipolar and primary unipolar affective disorder. Arch Gen Psychiatry 50:457–465, 1993b

Winokur G, Coryell W, Akiskal HS, et al: Manic-depressive (bipolar) disorder: the course in light of a prospective ten-year follow-up of 131 patients. Acta Psychiatr Scand 89:102–110, 1994

CHAPTER 14

Undertreatment of Major Depression

Robert Boland, M.D.
Martin B. Keller, M.D.
David Solomon, M.D.
Chunshan Li, M.A.
Andrew Leon, Ph.D.

DEPRESSION IS UNDERTREATED, despite the availability of effective treatments. This problem has been consistently observed for many decades (Weissman and Klerman 1977).

The Collaborative Depression Study (CDS) offered an opportunity to closely observe the treatment of depression. As this was an observational study, treatment was not influenced by the investigators. However, it was monitored with information provided by patients, relatives, medical records, and treatment staff.

Treatment was first examined in 1982 for the first 217 subjects who entered the study (Keller et al. 1982). The subjects included were those who had had major depressive disorder (MDD) for at least 1 month before entry into the study. Most patients were receiving either a tricyclic antidepressant (TCA) or a monoamine oxidase inhibitor (MAOI). Equivalent dose ranges were established to assess the adequacy of treatment, and information on other psychoactive treatments, including lithium or electroconvulsive therapy (ECT) and psychotherapy, received during the index episode also was recorded.

Treatment intensity was scored on a five-point scale, which ranged from 0 (no treatment) to 4 (use of a TCA, an MAOI, or lithium at a maximally effective dose for at least 4 weeks, or use of ECT) (Table 14–1).

Prior to study intake, the most commonly received treatments were psychotherapy (67%) or antianxiety medications (benzodiazepines) (55%). Only 34% of the patients studied received antidepressant medication for at least 4 consecutive weeks. In addition, only 12% of patients were receiving an adequate dose of medication (>150 mg of imipramine or its equivalent), and only 3% of the patients studied received medications at a maximally effective dose (at least 250 mg of imipramine or its equivalent for a minimum of 4 weeks). Of the 86 patients receiving antidepressant medication for at least 4 weeks, two-thirds received a lower and likely ineffective dose.

Surprisingly few variables were associated with intensity of treatment. Among sociodemographic variables, only age predicted that older patients were more likely to receive antianxiety medications. Patients with psychotic depression were more likely to receive intensive treatment, which is use of antipsychotic drugs and ECT. However, only 25% of the patients with psychotic depression received the most intensive treatment (a maximum dose of an antidepressant, plus an antipsychotic or ECT). The duration of the episode prior to intake did not predict treatment intensity nor did a history of one or more suicide attempts.

The CDS investigators concluded that they were "surprised and concerned" by the small proportion of patients who were receiving adequate treatment. Although the reasons for this undertreatment were unknown, they speculated that factors related to both patients and caregivers were likely important. They noted that many patients delayed seeking treatment because of a failure to recognize the illness and a fear of stigmatization. This may have led patients to avoid or not comply with treatment. In addition, clinicians may have failed to recognize a depressive disorder, underestimated its severity, been unaware of optimal treatments, underestimated the effectiveness of treatment, or overestimated the risk for side effects. Given the high prevalence of mood disorders, this inadequacy of treatment, despite information and education on the recognition and treatment of depression, was deemed a significant public health concern.

Reactions to the Collaborative Depression Study Findings

Although many clinicians shared this concern about undertreatment, some took issue with the findings. Several editorials that accompanied the original article suggested that there may be good reasons for physician reluctance to

TABLE 14–1. Composite antidepressant score

Score	Amounts and combinations of somatic therapies
0	No treatment
1	Any imipramine, MAOI, 1 ECT, or alprazolam; or 1,000 mg of tryptophan or more; but less than:
2	100 mg of imipramine or 30 mg of MAOI, or more; or any lithium carbonate; or 3,000 mg of tryptophan or more; but less than:
3	200 mg of imipramine or 60 mg of MAOI or 2 ECT, or more; but less than:
4	300 mg of imipramine or 75 mg of MAOI or 3 ECT, or more

Note. ECT=electroconvulsive therapy (number of treatments per week); MAOI= monoamine oxidase inhibitor.

prescribe antidepressants and patient reluctance to take them. Lundberg (1982) cited concerns about the toxicity of antidepressants and their potential to increase suicide risk. Uhlenhuth (1982) alluded to the long time to response, the difficulty in achieving proper doses, the substantial side effects of TCAs and MAOIs, and their potential lethality in suicide attempts. When considering this against the conflicting data regarding the efficacy and specificity of psychotropic medications, he argued that the CDS findings might reflect a rational consideration of the risk-benefit ratio by physicians.

Subsequent Prospective Data on the Adequacy of Treatment

This first study examined only treatment that was given prior to intake to the CDS. The first prospective analysis of treatment in the CDS cohort was in 1986 (Keller et al. 1986a) and reported on 338 patients with MDD during their first 8 weeks after entry into the study. Once in the study, the intensity of treatment increased. However, treatment intensity generally remained inadequate: of those entering the study as inpatients, 31% received either no antidepressant treatment or only low levels, and only 49% received intensive therapy for 4 weeks. Of those entering as outpatients, 29% received no antidepressant medications, 24% had low levels of treatment, and only 19% received intensive treatment (a maximum therapeutic dose for 4 weeks of the study). Psychotherapy also was underused: 19% of the inpatients and 52% of the outpatients received less than 30 minutes of psychotherapy per week. The intensity of treatment varied across the different centers of the study; however, these differences in treatment were not predicted by the clinical variables. Given the importance of the study center and the limited association of sociodemographic or clinical variables, the authors suggested that the typically low level of treatment observed was attributable to differences in clinicians' approaches to treatment and concluded that "we are concerned that the actual patient in the clinician's practice may be treated more capriciously and less well than the theoretical patient in the clinician's textbooks" (Keller et al. 1986a, p. 466).

Again, interpretations differed. In an accompanying commentary, Kupfer and Freedman (1986) noted that the CDS was not designed to answer the relevant questions raised because one cannot know from the observational data why the treating clinicians made particular decisions. They suggested that it might be possible in the future to understand not only the treatments given but also the rationale behind treatment decisions, without influencing the decisions, but that contemporary data shed little light on this question.

Although the reasons for undertreatment were not clear, it seems meaningful that 67% of the patients seen at 8 weeks had not yet recovered from their index episode, highlighting the consequences of inadequate treatment. This trend continued as the study progressed: 50% of patients who were depressed for 2 years or longer after entry into the study received no or minimal somatic treatment (Keller et al. 1984). Among patients who recovered from an episode of depression and then had a recurrence, 50% had not received maintenance treatment in the month before the recurrence (Keller et al. 1983), and 60% of patients who had a recurrence and then remained depressed for longer than a year received little or no treatment (Keller et al. 1986b).

Corroboration From Other Studies

Several other studies conducted during the same period also reported inadequate treatment, particularly in the primary care setting. For example, one study reported that a significant number of primary care physicians both misdiagnose and undertreat depression (Perez-Stable et al. 1990). Another study found that only half of the depressed patients receiving treatment in a primary care clinic were given treatment for depression (Simon and VonKorff 1995). A third study (Katon et al. 1992) similarly found that approximately half of patients treated in primary care settings received antidepressants, and only 11% received adequate doses and durations of treatment. The Medical Outcomes Study (Wells et al. 1989) reported that psychiatrists were the most likely to prescribe antidepressants for patients with MDD. Even then, only about one-third of the patients with depression were given treatment, and of those, fewer than one-half received adequate treatment.

The National Depressive and Manic-Depressive Association Consensus Statement on the Undertreatment of Depression

In response to concerns raised by these and other findings, the National Depressive and Manic-Depressive Association (NDMDA) organized a consensus conference on the undertreatment of depression in 1996 (Hirschfeld et al. 1997). The expert panel concluded that overwhelming evidence indicated that depression was seriously undertreated despite the availability of safe and effective treatments. The cost of this undertreatment to society and individuals was considered substantial and resulted in suffering, social and occupational impairment, and suicide. Reasons for this undertreatment were considered and were thought to involve patient, provider, and health care system factors. Patient factors included a failure to recognize symptoms of the disorder, a tendency to underestimate the severity of the symptoms, limited access to health care, stigma, noncompliance, and economic factors. Provider factors included a lack of education about depression, limited training and time for detecting these symptoms, stigma, and a tendency to undertreat with medications and neglect psychotherapeutic approaches. Health care, including mental health care, systems also contained barriers, particularly economic disincentives to seeking and receiving adequate health care. The conference suggested several strategies to narrow the gap between knowledge and practice, including enhancing the role of patients and families, developing performance standards for behavioral health care systems, introducing incentives for proper assessment and treatment of depression, enhancing education programs, and continuing to research improved treatments for depression.

Recent Findings on Continued Undertreatment

The past decade has brought some advances in the treatment of depression. The attention fostered by efforts such as the NDMDA conference and other organizations has helped to increase awareness and decrease the potential stigma surrounding this disorder. Most medical schools have greatly increased the education devoted to the evaluation and treatment of mental disorders. The publication of treatment algorithms such as the Texas Medication Algorithm Project (Ereshefsky 2001) and the availability of practice guidelines such as those of the American Psychiatric Association (McIntyre 2001) or the National Institute for Health and Clinical Excellence in the United Kingdom (NICE; Clark 2011) have helped to disseminate a standard of care. Perhaps most important, the addition of newer antidepressants (e.g., selective serotonin reuptake inhibitors and serotonin-norepinephrine reuptake inhibitors) has simplified treatment by introducing agents that are better tolerated by patients and simpler to dose. One would assume that now that adequate dosing is simpler to achieve, more patients would receive treatment.

In the wake of these advances, is undertreatment of depression still a challenge? Discouragingly, it appears that the undertreatment of depression remains a significant challenge. The National Institute of Mental Health–sponsored REVAMP (Research Evaluating the Value of Augmentation of Medication by Psychotherapy) trial in 2008 found that only 33% of the 801 subjects enrolled (from 2002 to 2006) with chronic major depression had ever had a prior adequate trial of antidepressant medication (Kocsis et al. 2008). This result is similar to the rates reported by the earlier studies mentioned in this chapter.

These results are remarkably similar to the final summary results from the CDS. In examining the data for the entire 30 years of the study, we analyzed data on patients who experienced at least one episode of depression prospectively observed during the period of the study, looking at treatment given both during weeks that an individual experienced MDD and during weeks in which the person was well. We found that somatic treatment (defined as the use of any antidepressant, lithium, or ECT) was given only 57% of the time during weeks in which a patient was depressed and only 37% of the time during well weeks, despite the fact that the illness was highly recurrent in most patients.

Although the CDS did not collect sufficient data to evaluate the adequacy of psychotherapy treatment, evidence suggests that this treatment is underused as well in both primary care (Stafford et al. 2000) and psychiatric (Cully et al. 2008) settings. Evidence, albeit from a decade ago, suggested that when patients do present for treatment, their symptoms are managed with pharmacotherapy alone (Olfson et al. 2002). For example, in one survey of patients with anxiety or depression (recruited through treatment advocacy groups), 88% reported having had medications recommended to them, but only 39% were recommended to begin psychotherapy (Wang et al. 2000). Little evidence suggests that this situation has improved over the past decade (Collins et al. 2004), and in the context of current health care funding challenges, the problem will likely worsen.

These findings on the undertreatment of depression should be considered in the larger context of the problem of the undertreatment of common and treatable medical illnesses in general. The U.S. Food and Drug Administration (2012) has characterized this as a "well recognized public health problem," and good evidence supports this concern. Common and potentially preventable diseases such as hyperlipidemia (Verma et al. 2012), hypertension (Wu and Gerstenblith 2010), migraine headaches (Bigal et al. 2009), type 2 diabetes (Kones 2011), asthma (Fuhrman et al. 2011), and chronic obstructive pulmonary disease (Make et al. 2012) are all reported to be insufficiently treated, often despite comprehensive educational efforts.

Conclusion and Future Directions

Thus, the problem of undertreating depression remains a stubborn one. The many efforts to improve treatment, including various public health initiatives and patient- and clinician-centered education efforts, have not significantly improved the situation nor have the many improvements and additions to our somatotherapy arsenal. The explanation for this continues to be perplexing, but it is reasonable to assume that the dissenting opinions expressed by some experts in their critiques of the data account for some of the reticence to use available treatments. Antidepressants still may be seen as an inadequate solution to the problem of depression in that, despite improvements, they continue to have significant limitations. These criticisms are understandable given the ongoing published concerns about their tolerability (Clayton 2012).

Although currently available somatotherapies for depression do have limitations, coupled with various psychotherapies, they remain the best treatments available (Keller et al. 2000). Given the immense burden of untreated major depression, we continue to believe that the undertreatment of depression is a significant yet potentially resolvable problem. More work must be done to understand the nature of this problem. In the meantime, efforts to educate, influence, and perhaps mandate the use of intensive treatment for major depression should be a priority of future preventive mental health care efforts. Ultimately, we may have to rely on the art and the science of medicine. Treatment guidelines and education can only do so much, and we must rely on the skill of the clinician to create the sort of trusting therapeutic relationship that is necessary for successful treatment.

Clinical Implications

- Despite efforts to educate clinicians and the public, and the availability of safe and effective treatments, depression is still seriously undertreated.

- The cost of undertreatment in terms of patient suffering and loss of income is substantial.
- The reasons for this undertreatment are likely multifactorial, involving patient, provider, and health care system factors. Currently, efforts to address these factors have not significantly changed the rate of undertreatment.
- Undertreatment in part may reflect continued skepticism about the adequacy of current treatments as well as the risk of adverse effects.
- Despite their limitations, antidepressants, coupled with psychotherapy, remain the best available treatments for this very disabling disorder.

References

Bigal M, Krymchantowski AV, Lipton RB: Barriers to satisfactory migraine outcomes: what have we learned, where do we stand? Headache 49:1028–1041, 2009

Clark DM: Implementing NICE guidelines for the psychological treatment of depression and anxiety disorders: the IAPT experience. Int Rev Psychiatry 23:318–327, 2011

Clayton AH: Understanding antidepressant mechanism of action and its effect on efficacy and safety. J Clin Psychiatry 73:e11, 2012

Collins KA, Westra HA, Dozois DJ, et al: Gaps in accessing treatment for anxiety and depression: challenges for the delivery of care. Clin Psychol Rev 24:583–616, 2004

Cully JA, Tolpin L, Jimenez D, et al: Psychotherapy in the Veterans Health Administration: missed opportunities? Psychol Serv 55:320–331, 2008

Ereshefsky L: The Texas Medication Algorithm Project for major depression. Manag Care 10 (8 suppl):16–17; discussion 18–22, 2001

Fuhrman C, Dubus JC, Marguet C, et al: Hospitalizations for asthma in children are linked to undertreatment and insufficient asthma education. J Asthma 48:565–571, 2011

Hirschfeld RM, Keller MB, Panico S, et al: The National Depressive and Manic-Depressive Association consensus statement on the undertreatment of depression. JAMA 277:333–340, 1997

Katon W, von Korff M, Lin E, et al: Adequacy and duration of antidepressant treatment in primary care. Med Care 30:67–76, 1992

Keller MB, Klerman GL, Lavori PW, et al: Treatment received by depressed patients. JAMA 248:1848–1855, 1982

Keller MB, Lavori PW, Lewis CE, et al: Predictors of relapse in major depressive disorder. JAMA 250:3299–3304, 1983

Keller MB, Klerman GL, Lavori PW, et al: Long-term outcome of episodes of major depression: clinical and public health significance. JAMA 252:788–792, 1984

Keller MB, Lavori PW, Klerman GL, et al: Low levels and lack of predictors of somato-therapy and psychotherapy received by depressed patients. Arch Gen Psychiatry 43:458–466, 1986a

Keller MB, Lavori PW, Rice J, et al: The persistent risk of chronicity in recurrent episodes of nonbipolar major depressive disorder: a prospective follow-up. Am J Psychiatry 143:24–28, 1986b

Keller MB, McCullough JP, Klein DN, et al: A comparison of nefazodone, the cognitive behavioral-analysis system of psychotherapy, and their combination for the treatment of chronic depression. N Engl J Med 342:1462–1470, 2000

Kocsis JH, Gelenberg AJ, Rothbaum B, et al: Chronic forms of major depression are still undertreated in the 21st century: systematic assessment of 801 patients presenting for treatment. J Affect Disord 110:55–61, 2008

Kones R: Is prevention a fantasy, or the future of medicine? A panoramic view of recent data, status, and direction in cardiovascular prevention. Ther Adv Cardiovasc Dis 5:61–81, 2011

Kupfer DJ, Freedman DX: Treatment for depression: 'standard' clinical practice as an unexamined topic. Arch Gen Psychiatry 43:509–511, 1986

Lundberg GD: Antidepressive drugs as a cause of death. JAMA 248:1879, 1982

Make B, Dutro MP, Paulose-Ram R, et al: Undertreatment of COPD: a retrospective analysis of US managed care and Medicare patients. Int J Chron Obstruct Pulmon Dis 7:1–9, 2012

McIntyre JS: Depression and practice guidelines. Hum Psychopharmacol 16:115–118, 2001

Olfson M, Marcus SC, Druss B, et al: National trends in the outpatient treatment of depression. JAMA 287:203–209, 2002

Perez-Stable EJ, Miranda J, Munoz RF, et al: Depression in medical outpatients: underrecognition and misdiagnosis. Arch Intern Med 150:1083–1088, 1990

Simon GE, VonKorff M: Recognition, management, and outcomes of depression in primary care. Arch Fam Med 4:99–105, 1995

Stafford RS, Ausiello JC, Misra B, et al: National patterns of depression treatment in primary care. Prim Care Companion J Clin Psychiatry 2:211–216, 2000

Uhlenhuth EH: Depressives, doctors, and antidepressants. JAMA 248:1879–1880, 1982

U.S. Food and Drug Administration: FDA considers expanding definition of nonprescription drugs. March 23, 2012. Available at: www.fda.gov/Drugs/ResourcesForYou/SpecialFeatures/ucm297128.htm. Accessed August 23, 2012.

Verma A, Visintainer P, Elarabi M, et al: Overtreatment and undertreatment of hyperlipidemia in the outpatient setting. South Med J 105:329–333, 2012

Wang PS, Berglund P, Kessler RC: Recent care of common mental disorders in the United States: prevalence and conformance with evidence-based recommendations. J Gen Intern Med 15:284–292, 2000

Weissman MM, Klerman GL: The chronic depressive in the community: unrecognized and poorly treated. Compr Psychiatry 18:523–532, 1977

Wells KB, Stewart A, Hays RD, et al: The functioning and well-being of depressed patients: results from the Medical Outcomes Study. JAMA 262:914–919, 1989

Wu KC, Gerstenblith G: Update on newer antihypertensive medicines and interventions. J Cardiovasc Pharmacol Ther 15:257–267, 2010

CHAPTER 15

Impact of Anxiety Severity on Mood Disorders

Jan A. Fawcett, M.D.

William H. Coryell, M.D.

Paula Clayton, M.D.

IT HAS BEEN CUSTOMARY to separate mood disorders from anxiety disorders as diagnostic categories, and no previous edition of the American Psychiatric Association's *Diagnostic and Statistical Manual of Mental Disorders* (DSM) has considered the presence of anxiety symptoms when subtyping mood disorders.

Beginning with the Collaborative Depression Study (CDS), numerous studies have examined the presence, severity, and role of anxiety symptoms in the clinical outcome of mood disorders, both major depressive disorder and bipolar depression (e.g., Maser and Cloninger 1990). In this chapter, we review the findings of the CDS and of subsequent studies concerning the prognostic effects of anxiety on mood disorders, whether that anxiety is measured by the presence of comorbid anxiety disorders or by the severity of anxiety symptoms. The CDS data are particularly useful for this purpose because the Schedule for Affective Disorders and Schizophrenia (SADS; Endicott and Spitzer 1978; see Chapter 2, "Collaborative Depression Study Procedures and Study Design") records the severity of symptoms as well as the presence or absence of individual symptoms and full anxiety syndromes. Therefore, we present research in which anxiety is measured by the presence of comorbid anxiety, the severity of anxiety symptoms, or both.

Overall et al. (1966) derived three and Paykel (1971) derived four subtypes of depression, of which the anxious/tense subtype was the largest group in each system. Clayton (1993) noted that these reports confirmed the association between anxious and agitated depression discussed by Sir Aubrey Lewis (1970). Studies that have compared patients with and without anxiety or panic symptoms generally have found that those with severe anxiety symptoms have more severe depressive disorders (Coryell et al. 2009, 2012; Fava et al. 2004, 2006; Fawcett and Kravitz 1983; Stordal et al. 2008) whether measured by the SADS-C (Change Version) Psychic Anxiety Scale (Clayton et al. 1991; Coryell et al. 2009, 2012; Fawcett and Kravitz 1983), the Hospital Depression Scale (Stordal et al. 2008), or the Hamilton Rating Scale for Depression Anxiety/Somatization subscale (Fava et al. 2004, 2006; Thase 2009).

Initial Findings From the Collaborative Depression Study on the Effect of Anxiety on Mood Disorders

In 1983, Fawcett and Kravitz characterized the presence and severity of anxiety symptoms as measured by the SADS-C Psychic Anxiety Scale. Results from 200 patients with major depressive episodes (MDEs)—mainly CDS patients from the recruitment site of Rush-Presbyterian-St. Luke's Hospital, Rush College of Medicine in Chicago—showed that 62% had psychic anxiety of at least moderate severity, whereas 38% had moderately severe to severe levels. With respect to worry, 72% admitted to worry of moderate severity (4 on a severity scale of 0–6), and 42% had severe worry (5 on a severity scale of 0–6). Somatic anxiety, defined as the presence of autonomic and muscular symptomatology and described by patients in terms of bodily sensations, was present to a moderate level in 42% of patients and to a moderately severe level in 21% of patients diagnosed by the Research Diagnostic Criteria (RDC) with an MDE. Panic attacks were present in 29%. Patients with an RDC endogenous MDE, a subtype of greater severity, had more severe anxiety than did those with nonendogenous depression.

In 1990, Fawcett et al. reported on 13 patients who had committed suicide within 1 year of entry into the CDS and another 19 who had done so 2–10 years after entry out of a sample of 954 patients with major affective disorders. A comparison of the short-term suicide patients with the 920 patients who survived found that the former had had significantly more severe psychic anxiety at baseline and were more likely to have been experiencing panic attacks than were the patients who did not commit suicide; however, standard risk factors such as severity of suicidal ideation, prior suicide attempts (past or recent), and severity of hopelessness were not predictive. In contrast, baseline hopelessness and suicidal ideation separated those who committed suicide after the first 12 months from those who did not, whereas psychic anxiety did not separate suicides from nonsuicides. This difference in the importance of baseline anxiety to short- but not long-term suicide persisted after the number of long-term suicides had increased to 25 patients (Maser et al. 2002).

Maser et al. (2002) compared the 14-year CDS records of 36 patients who committed suicide, 120 who attempted suicide, and 373 with no recorded suicide attempt. High scores on the two newly derived "impulsivity" factors, plus three additional personality items, significantly differentiated short-term suicide completers from comparison group patients. Risk of suicide within 1 year of evaluation increased if the patient had clinically significant psychic anxiety, panic attacks, emotional turmoil plus depression or cycling/mixed affective syndromes, or delusions of mind reading or thought insertion in the index episode. Risk of early suicide also was increased as a function of current or past substance abuse, antisocial personality, and absence of children age 18 or younger in the home at the time of study intake.

In 1991, Clayton et al. summed the severity of six anxiety symptoms in 320 patients with primary major depression. They found a high frequency of anxiety symptoms across the sample, and a small proportion (<10%) had very high summed anxiety scale scores. Severity of anxiety symptoms correlated with poor outcome over 10 years and with a family history of depression but not of panic disorder.

Two analyses of CDS data considered relations between baseline anxiety levels based on SADS anxiety symptom severity and subsequent long-term morbidity as measured by the proportion of weeks in mood disorder episodes (Coryell et al. 2009, 2012). A strong linear relation existed between the baseline severity of anxiety measures and the proportions of time spent over the following 16–20 years in periods of depression ($P = 0.001$), although no relation was seen between baseline anxiety severity and time spent in periods of mania or hypomania (see Figure 1 in Coryell et al. 2009). The relation showed little diminution over 25 years (Coryell et al. 2012), an indication that a high level of anxiety accompanying an MDE identifies a stable quality of the illness rather than only of the depressive episode.

Relevant Research Findings From Other Studies Published Recently and Newer Collaborative Depression Study Findings

In 2007, Simon et al. described a merged managed care database of 32,000 bipolar patients and found that a comorbid diagnosis of generalized anxiety disorder, panic disorder, or anxiety disorder not otherwise specified significantly increased the likelihood of suicide (odds ratio [OR] = 1.4) or suicide attempts (OR = 1.2). This study presented the frequency of comorbid anxiety disorder diagnosis but not the severity of the anxiety experienced by the patients.

Stordal et al. (2008) studied 10,670 male and 3,883 female suicides from a sample of 60,000 Norwegian citizens who completed the Hospital Anxiety and Depression Scale monthly, except for July, from 1995 to 1997. A correlation emerged between monthly variations in suicide rates and monthly variations in comorbid anxiety and depression ($r = 0.72$; $P = 0.01$). A significant monthly variation in the prevalence of depression ($P = 0.001$) but no monthly variation in the prevalence of anxiety occurred, suggesting that those with high anxiety experienced constant high levels, whereas depression varied in severity, conferring highest risk for suicide when reaching severe levels in these high-anxiety individuals.

Fava et al. (2004, 2006) used the Anxiety subscale of the Hamilton Rating Scale for Depression and found that those with higher anxiety severity scores had significantly lower response rates to treatment in the Sequenced Treatment Alternatives to Relieve Depression (STAR*D) study. Thase (2009) analyzed data from treatment phase 2 of the STAR*D study, in which patients failing to attain remission after taking citalopram were randomly assigned by clinical equipoise to five different treatments—namely, sertraline, venlafaxine, bupropion, and citalopram augmentation by buspirone or bupropion. Subjects with high levels of comorbid anxiety as determined by a median split were one-third to one-half as likely to respond to treatment as were those in the low-anxiety group.

In 2003, Busch et al. studied 76 patients who committed suicide while hospitalized or within a few days of hospital discharge. After chart review with the SADS-C Psychic Anxiety Scale, 79% were found to have had either increased anxiety or increased agitation during the week before their suicides.

In 2009, Pfeiffer et al. reported on suicide among 887,859 veterans with major depression and showed that patients with a comorbid diagnosis of generalized anxiety disorder, anxiety disorder not otherwise specified, or panic disorder had an elevated odds ratio (1.2–1.3) for suicide. Of particular interest was that patients taking the anxiolytics benzodiazepines and buspirone had an elevated odds ratio (1.7) for suicide and that the risk was even higher within a smaller sample of patients receiving high-dose anxiolytics (OR = 2.2). This treatment-dosage correlation suggests that in this study, the severity of comorbid anxiety seems related to suicide in patients with major depression. It also raises the possibility that the inhibition produced by high benzodiazepine doses may increase the likelihood of completed suicide.

This review of the relation of comorbid anxiety to poor therapeutic outcomes or suicide supports the theory that severity of anxious symptoms is related to these negative outcomes. Notably, others have shown in bipolar patients that increased anxiety levels are associated with greater impulsiveness (Taylor et al. 2008).

Conclusion

Goldberg and Fawcett (2012) reviewed some of the studies discussed earlier as well as epidemiological studies to emphasize the clinical importance of anxiety in both the bipolar and related disorders and depressive disorders chapters. The anxiety severity dimension proposed for use in both the bipolar and related disorders and the depressive disorders chapters in DSM-5 may focus more clinical attention on treating comorbid anxiety in patients with mood disorders. This proposal rests on the data reviewed earlier and reflects findings from the CDS and subsequent studies. Findings from the CDS have contributed to the growing recognition of the importance of anxiety symptoms across the mood disorders.

At this point, limited evidence exists for the effectiveness of treatment for anxiety symptoms that accompany mood disorders, although studies with aripiprazole and quetiapine have produced some evidence for this (Lydiard et al. 2009; McIntyre et al. 2007; Trivedi et al. 2008). It is hoped that further recognition of the significance for treatment outcome and the risk of suicide associated with severe anxiety symptoms in mood disorders will lead to more effective treatment.

Clinical Implications

- Anxiety severity is both common in major depression and predictive of negative outcomes.
- Anxiety symptoms are correlated with suicide over the initial weeks and months (up to 1 year of follow-up) and with a signif-

icantly higher presence of major depression over five successive
5-year follow-ups.

- Anxiety symptoms are associated with poorer treatment response in patients with mood disorders.
- The presence of severe anxiety symptoms is an important issue
in the management of mood disorders. On the basis of the previously discussed evidence, a quantitative rating of severity of
anxiety will be added to the diagnoses of mood disorders in
DSM-5 (see Chapter 16, "Contributions of the NIMH Collaborative Depression Study to DSM-5").

References

Busch KA, Fawcett J, Jacobs D: Clinical correlates of inpatient suicide. J Clin Psychiatry 64:14–19, 2003

Clayton P: Suicide in panic disorder and depression. Curr Ther Res Clin Exp 54:825–
831, 1993

Clayton PJ, Grove WM, Coryell W, et al: Follow-up and family study of anxious depression. Am J Psychiatry 148:1512–1517, 1991

Coryell W, Solomon DA, Fiedorowicz JG, et al: Anxiety and outcome in bipolar disorder. Am J Psychiatry 166:1238–1243, 2009

Coryell W, Fiedorowicz JG, Solomon D, et al: Effects of anxiety on the long-term
course of depressive disorders. Br J Psychiatry 200:210–215, 2012

Endicott J, Spitzer RL: A diagnostic interview: the Schedule for Affective Disorders
and Schizophrenia. Arch Gen Psychiatry 35:837–844, 1978

Fava M, Alpert JE, Carmin CN, et al: Clinical correlates and symptom patterns of anxious depression among patients with major depressive disorder in STAR*D. Psychol Med 34:1299–1308, 2004

Fava M, Rush AJ, Alpert JE, et al: What clinical and symptom features and comorbid
disorders characterize patients with anxious major depression in STAR*D? Can J
Psychiatry 51:823–835, 2006

Fawcett J, Kravitz HM: Anxiety symptoms and their relationship to depressive illness.
J Clin Psychiatry 44:8–11, 1983

Fawcett J, Scheftner WA, Fogg L, et al: Time-related predictors of suicide in major affective disorder. Am J Psychiatry 147:1189–1194, 1990

Goldberg D, Fawcett J: The importance of anxiety in both major depression and bipolar disorder. Depress Anxiety 29:1–8, 2012

Lewis A: The ambiguous word "anxiety." Int J Psychiatry 9:21–69, 1970

Lydiard RB, Culpepper L, Schiöler H, et al: Quetiapine monotherapy as treatment for
anxiety symptoms with bipolar depression: a pooled analysis of results from 2
double-blind, randomized, placebo-controlled trials. Prim Care Companion J Clin
Psychiatry 11:215–225, 2009

Maser JD, Cloninger CR (eds): Comorbidity of Mood and Anxiety Disorders. Washington, DC, American Psychiatric Press, 1990

Maser JD, Akiskal HS, Schettler P, et al: Can temperament identify affectively ill patients who engage in lethal or near-lethal suicidal behavior? A 14-year prospective study. Suicide Life Threat Behav 32:10–32, 2002

McIntyre A, Gendron A, McIntyre A: Quetiapine adjunct to selective serotonin reuptake inhibitors or venlafaxine in patients with major depression, comorbid anxiety, and residual depressive symptoms: a randomized, placebo controlled pilot study. Depress Anxiety 24:487–494, 2007

Overall JE, Hollister LE, Johnson M, et al: Nosology of depression and differential response to drugs. JAMA 195:946–948, 1966

Paykel ES: Classification of depressed patients: a cluster analysis derived grouping. Br J Psychiatry 118:275–288, 1971

Pfeiffer PN, Ganoczy D, Ilgen M, et al: Comorbid anxiety as a suicide risk factor among depressed veterans. Depress Anxiety 26:752–757, 2009

Simon GE, Hunkeler E, Fireman B, et al: Risk of suicide attempt and suicide death in patients treated for bipolar disorder. Bipolar Disord 9:526–530, 2007

Stordal E, Morken G, Mykletun A, et al: Monthly variation in prevalence rates of comorbid depression and anxiety in the general population at 63–65 degrees North: the Hunt study. J Affect Disord 103:273–278, 2008

Taylor CT, Hirshfeld-Becker DR, Ostacher MJ, et al: Anxiety is associated with impulsivity in bipolar disorder. J Anxiety Disord 22:868–876, 2008

Thase M: Update on partial response in depression. J Clin Psychiatry 70 (suppl 6):4–9, 2009

Trivedi MH, Thase ME, Fava M, et al: Adjunctive aripiprazole in major depressive disorder: analysis of safety and efficacy in patients with anxious and atypical features. J Clin Psychiatry 69:1928–1936, 2008

Contributions of the NIMH Collaborative Depression Study to DSM-5

Jan A. Fawcett, M.D.

DSM-5 EVOLVED from DSM-III (American Psychiatric Association 1980) through DSM-III-R, DSM-IV, and DSM-IV-TR (American Psychiatric Association 1987, 1994, 2000). DSM-III was a major departure from prior diagnostic systems reflected in DSM-I and DSM-II (American Psychiatric Association 1952, 1968), which tended to be highly influenced by theoretical thinking of the day. DSM-III was developed from the Research Diagnostic Criteria (RDC; Spitzer et al. 1978) and built on the Feighner criteria (Feighner et al. 1972). The Collaborative Depression Study (CDS) recorded RDC diagnoses based on information from the Schedule for Affective Disorders and Schizophrenia (SADS; Endicott and Spitzer 19789, 1979). The SADS was a unique clinical research instrument in that it did not limit symptom coverage to predetermined diagnostic categories, and it covered a range of symptoms and quantified the severity of the symptoms. This required the establishment not only of categorical diagnostic reliability but also of symptom severity reliability across the clinical raters. The RDC aggregated symptoms measured into categories, including an undiagnosed category, whereas the SADS allowed for the possibility of a severity spectrum of disorders, which will be reflected in DSM-5. This is a beginning of an attempt to address the heterogeneity of categorical diagnoses and the high rates of overlapping comorbid diagnoses.

A Spectrum View of Mood Disorders: The Mixed Specifier

An early report from the CDS (Akiskal et al. 1995) showed that over a follow-up period of 11 years, 8.6% of SADS-diagnosed "unipolar" depressed patients converted to bipolar II disorder, and 3.9% converted to bipolar I disorder. Another 5-year follow-up of 248 patients diagnosed with major depressive episode found that a total of 11.7% switched to bipolar diagnoses (8.2% bipolar II and 2.9% bipolar I) (Holma et al. 2008). More recently, Angst et al. (2011), in the Bridge study of 5,635 patients with DSM-IV major depressive episode, found a high proportion of patients with subthreshold hypomanic symptoms (31%) who resembled bipolar subjects in having family histories of bipolar disorder (odds ratio > 2; $P=0.001$) and multiple past mood episodes.

A much more recent CDS report on 550 patients with major depressive disorder (MDD) at intake who were followed up for a mean of 17.6 years (Fiedorowicz et al. 2011) indicated a total switch rate of 19.7%: 12.2% of patients to hypomania and 7.5% to mania. This study found that those patients who "switched" diagnoses were more likely to have several subthreshold manic symptoms, the presence of psychosis, an early age at onset, and a family history of bipolar disorder. This finding and another recent CDS analysis of subsyndromal bipolar symptoms in bipolar depressed patients (Judd et al. 2012) have influenced the proposal for a mixed specifier across both unipolar MDD and bipolar disorders in DSM-5. This is particularly important because studies have pointed to the possibility that antidepressant medications worsen not only the course of bipolar disorder but also that of MDD with mixed features. Several studies have also questioned the effectiveness of antidepressant medications, including tricyclic antidepressants, selective serotonin reuptake inhibitors, serotonin-norepinephrine reuptake inhibitors, and bupropion, in the treatment of depression in bipolar patients (Sachs et al. 2007; Sidor and MacQueen 2011).

A unique change in DSM-5 will be to eliminate the diagnosis of bipolar I disorder, mixed type, which required that the patient simultaneously meet full criteria for MDD and mania. DSM-5 will instead have a mixed specifier across MDD and the bipolar spectrum (bipolar I, II) that will note the presence of at least three depressive symptoms in manic or hypomanic patients or at least three manic symptoms (e.g., grandiosity, racing/crowded thoughts, increased energy, and goal-directed activity but not irritability) in patients with

MDD. This should help the clinician to diagnose mixed features across mood disorders and not limit the mixed designation to those meeting full bipolar I criteria. It will also flag the presence of manic symptoms in those with MDD.

Importance of Severe Anxiety Comorbidity in Mood Disorders

The first CDS report of the high frequency of anxiety symptoms in MDD was published in 1983 (Fawcett and Kravitz 1983); 63% of the patients with major depression had at least a moderate severity of anxiety symptoms, and in 38%, they were severe. Moderate worry was found in 72%, severe worry in 42%, and panic attacks in 29%.

A 10-year follow-up of CDS patients found that severe comorbid psychic anxiety, severe global insomnia, and the occurrence of panic attacks increased the risk of suicide in the first year of follow-up, and standard suicide risk factors such as prior attempts (past or recent), severity of hopelessness, and severity of suicidal ideation showed a significant association later in the follow-up period (Fawcett et al. 1990). Clayton et al. (1991) reported on a subset of 320 patients from the CDS sample with primary MDD (implying the absence of a prior nonaffective diagnosis, including any anxiety disorder). They found a high frequency of anxiety symptoms by summing the severity scores of six subscales of various measures of anxiety (i.e., somatic anxiety, panic attacks, psychic anxiety, agitation, worry) from total severity scales at baseline entry into the study. They also found that the patients with the most severe levels of summed anxiety scores had the worst treatment outcomes and stronger family history of major depression but not panic disorders.

Subsequent retrospective findings of Hall et al. (1999) supported the relevance of anxiety on clinical outcomes in those with mood disorders; of 100 patients admitted from an emergency department for a suicide attempt and interviewed with the SADS-C (Change Version), 90% reported severe levels of psychic anxiety for 1 month before their attempt. This was a partial replication of the CDS finding that high severe anxiety was associated with the risk of suicide over a 1-year period.

Data from the Sequenced Treatment Alternatives to Relieve Depression (STAR*D) study by Fava et al. (2004, 2006) found that slightly fewer than half of the 2,876 patients with unipolar major depression treated with citalopram in Level I of the study had severe comorbid anxiety, as measured by a subscale of anxiety, agitation, and somatic symptoms from the Hamilton Rating Scale for Depression, and that those patients with comorbid high anxiety had poorer responses to treatment. Another, later, report from the Systematic

Treatment Enhancement Program for Bipolar Disorder (STEP-BD) study (Simon 2009) found that bipolar patients with comorbid anxiety disorders had higher rates of disability, impairment, and suicidality.

Simon et al. (2007) described 32,000 patients with bipolar disorders in a managed care cohort. Those with comorbid generalized anxiety disorder had a significantly elevated odds of suicide and suicide attempts, whereas a comorbid diagnosis of substance use disorders was associated with a significantly higher odds of only suicide attempts but not suicide. Stordal et al. (2008) studied a sample of 10,670 males and 3,700 females who committed suicide and found a significant positive correlation ($r=0.0.72$; $P=0.01$) between the national suicide rate and the monthly variation in comorbid anxiety and depression.

Pfeiffer et al. (2009) found a significantly elevated odds ratio (1.3) for suicide among 887,859 veterans receiving treatment for depression with comorbid generalized anxiety disorder, anxiety disorder not otherwise specified, and panic disorder but not in those with other comorbid anxiety disorders, including post-traumatic stress disorder. Patients taking benzodiazepines and buspirone had a significantly elevated odds ratio (1.7) for suicide, and those taking high-dose anxiolytics had an even higher odds ratio (2.3) for suicide. This latter finding again suggests the importance of anxiety severity as a correlate of suicide.

More recently, Coryell et al. (2009, 2012) used CDS data to report that baseline comorbid anxiety symptom severity (psychic anxiety, somatic anxiety) correlated with the duration of depression experienced throughout a 20-year follow-up period, a strong indicator of the importance of the severity of anxiety symptoms for long-term outcome in mood disorders.

On the basis of this evidence, an anxiety severity dimension will be rated in addition to the diagnosis of a mood disorder in DSM-5. This unique addition of an anxiety severity scale to categorical diagnoses derives from the early CDS findings of the clinical importance of comorbid anxiety for the outcome of mood disorders.

Suicide in the Collaborative Depression Study and DSM-5

Suicide is one of the most important adverse outcomes in psychiatry. It is the eleventh leading cause of death in the United States and has been the most common sentinel event reported by 24-hour medical care facilities to the Joint Commission of Hospitals since 1994 (The Joint Commission 2010).

In previous editions of the DSM, suicide is not listed in the index and is referred to only in the sense that suicidal ideation or behavior is a criterion for MDD, that it is unpredictable, and that suicidal behavior occurs commonly in borderline personality disorder and alcohol and substance abuse disorders

(American Psychiatric Association 1994, 2000). Little is mentioned of suicide risk factors, and a suicide assessment is not discussed.

In a study of suicides occurring in the CDS with a prospective follow-up, careful recording of the presence and severity of clinical symptoms permitted the first attempt to view the prospective risk of suicide in terms of acute and chronic risk factors. The CDS risk factors for suicide, including current psychomotor agitation, marked anxiety, and current feelings of hopelessness, were included in the list of current risk factors.

The concept of current acute risk factors, as well as the addition of severe anxiety or agitation as a potential treatment-modifiable risk factor, stems from the prospective study of suicide from the CDS. This is reflected by the scaled level of clinical concern for suicide risk assessment by the clinician that was proposed for inclusion in DSM-5. The clinician could have used the scale to record his or her judgment as to how much of the treatment plan would be devoted to the prevention of suicide at any point in the clinical assessment of the patient. The scale is worded in terms to avoid any suggestion that suicide is predictable in an individual because multiple efforts have shown that no scale has the capacity to accurately predict suicidal behavior in an individual patient (Pokorny 1993). A guide to clinical factors was derived from a literature review to include risk factors such as suicidal behavior in the distant past, recently (past 3 months—e.g., a major real or anticipated loss), or currently. This guide, together with the clinician's experience and current clinical evaluation, would determine to what extent the treatment plan would be directed toward the prevention of suicide in a specific patient, which would be reflected in the clinician's rating of concern for suicide on a scale of 0–4. This suicide assessment makes clear that no evidence indicates that predictive weight should be assigned to these factors, and, in fact, the appropriate weighting of these factors may vary from patient to patient, making this a qualitative list of risk factors rather than a quantitative risk scale. Assigning a concern for suicide level would encourage a more complete suicide assessment and provide evidence that the clinician made a thoughtful assessment even though suicide cannot be accurately predicted in an individual.

This assessment system was tested in the DSM-5 Field Trials for reliability of ratings by a second clinician with the assessment readministered to the same patient within 2 weeks. The assessment consisted of two components: 1) the list of 14 risk factors scored on a yes-or-no basis for the field trial and 2) the clinician's concern about suicide risk scored on a 5-point ordinal scale. The test-retest reliability of the scale (risk factor and the clinician's concern for suicide) was tested across seven adult DSM-5 Field Trial sites among 1,412 patients. The pooled intraclass correlation coefficient associated with the dimensional ratings of clinician's concern about suicide risk was 0.48 (95% confidence interval [CI] = 0.42–0.52). This intraclass correlation value and the associated 95% CI indicate acceptable reliability of the scale (Kraemer et al. 2012).

Clinical Implications

- Findings from the Collaborative Depression Study have cast more light on mixed features that occur across both unipolar and bipolar mood disorders, phenomena that appear to be important determinants of outcomes such as course of illness and treatment response.
- The severity of comorbid anxiety appears to be related to poor outcomes of treatment, and this finding should increase attention to the treatment of comorbid anxiety as well as to the development of more effective treatments for this problem.
- Severe psychic anxiety was shown to be a risk factor for acute suicide, and this modifiable risk factor has been included in the items the literature supports for suicide risk factors.
- Attention to and treatment targeted to severe anxiety and agitation may reduce the incidence of suicide by focusing clinical attention on this potentially modifiable risk factor.
- The addition of a suicide risk assessment scale in DSM that uses a literature-based guide to risk factors and the clinician's experience and clinical judgment could improve screening of key risk factors for suicide.

References

Akiskal HS, Maser JD, Zeller PJ, et al: Switching from 'unipolar' to bipolar II: an 11-year prospective study of clinical and temperamental predictors in 559 patients. Arch Gen Psychiatry 52:114–123, 1995

American Psychiatric Association: Diagnostic and Statistical Manual: Mental Disorders. Washington, DC, American Psychiatric Association, 1952

American Psychiatric Association: Diagnostic and Statistical Manual of Mental Disorders, 2nd Edition. Washington, DC, American Psychiatric Association, 1968

American Psychiatric Association: Diagnostic and Statistical Manual of Mental Disorders, 3rd Edition. Washington, DC, American Psychiatric Association, 1980

American Psychiatric Association: Diagnostic and Statistical Manual of Mental Disorders, 3rd Edition, Revised. Washington, DC, American Psychiatric Association, 1987

American Psychiatric Association: Diagnostic and Statistical Manual of Mental Disorders, 4th Edition. Washington, DC, American Psychiatric Association, 1994

American Psychiatric Association: Diagnostic and Statistical Manual of Mental Disorders, 4th Edition, Text Revision. Washington, DC, American Psychiatric Association, 2000

Angst J, Azorin JM, Bowden CL, et al: Prevalence and characteristics of undiagnosed bipolar disorders in patients with a major depressive episode: the Bridge study. Arch Gen Psychiatry 68:791–798, 2011

Clayton PJ, Grove WW, Coryell W, et al: Follow-up and family study of anxious depression. Am J Psychiatry 148:1512–1517, 1991

Coryell W, Solomon DA, Fiedorowicz JG, et al: Anxiety and outcome in bipolar disorder. Am J Psychiatry 166:1238–1243, 2009

Coryell W, Fiedorowicz JG, Solomon D: Effects of anxiety on the long-term course of depressive disorders. Br J Psychiatry 200:210–215, 2012

Endicott J, Spitzer RL: A diagnostic interview: the Schedule for Affective Disorders and Schizophrenia. Arch Gen Psychiatry 35:837–844, 1978

Endicott J, Spitzer RL: Use of Research Diagnostic Criteria and the Schedule for Affective Disorders and Schizophrenia to study affective disorders. Am J Psychiatry 136:52–56, 1979

Fava M, Alpert JE, Carmin N, et al: Clinical correlates and symptom patterns of anxious depression among patients with major depressive disorder in STAR*D. Psychol Med 34:1299–1308, 2004

Fava M, Rush AJ, Alpert JE, et al: What clinical and symptom features and comorbid disorders characterize patients with anxious major depression in STAR*D? Can J Psychiatry 51:823–835, 2006

Fawcett J, Kravitz HM: Anxiety symptoms and their relationship to psychiatric illness. J Clin Psychiatry 44:8–11, 1983

Fawcett J, Scheftner WA, Fogg L, et al: Time-related predictors of suicide in major affective disorder. Am J Psychiatry 147:1189–1194, 1990

Feighner JP, Robins E, Guze SR, et al: Diagnostic criteria for use in psychiatric research. Arch Gen Psychiatry 26:40–48, 1972

Fiedorowicz JG, Endicott J, Leon A, et al: Subthreshold hypomanic symptoms in progression from unipolar major depression to bipolar depression. Am J Psychiatry 168:40–48, 2011

Hall RC, Platt DE, Hall RC: Suicide risk assessment: a review of suicide risk in 100 patients who made severe suicide attempts: evaluation of suicide risk in a time of managed care. Psychosomatics 4:18–22, 1999

Holma KM, Melartin K, Holma IA, et al: Predictors for switch from unipolar major depressive disorder to bipolar disorder type I or II: a 5-year prospective study. J Clin Psychiatry 69:1267–1275, 2008

The Joint Commission: Sentinel Event Alert. Issue 46, November 17, 2010

Judd LL, Schettler PJ, Akiskal HS, et al: Prevalence and significance of subsyndromal symptoms, including irritability and psychomotor agitation, during bipolar major depressive episodes. J Affect Disord 138:440–448, 2012

Kraemer HC, Kupfer DJ, Clarke DE, et al: DSM-5: how reliable is reliable enough? Am J Psychiatry 169:13–15, 2012

Pfeiffer PN, Ganoczy D, Ilgen M, et al: Comorbid anxiety as a risk factor among depressed veterans. Depress Anxiety 26:752–757, 2009

Pokorny AD: Suicide prediction revisited. Suicide Life Threat Behav 23:1–10, 1993

Sachs GS, Nierenberg AA, Calabrese JR, et al: Effectiveness of adjunctive antidepressant treatment for bipolar depression. N Engl J Med 356:1711–1722, 2007

Sidor MM, MacQueen GM: Antidepressants for the acute treatment of bipolar depression: a systematic review and meta-analysis. J Clin Psychiatry 72:156–157, 2011

Simon GE, Hunkeler E, Fireman B, et al: Risk of suicide attempt and suicide death in patients treated for bipolar disorder. Bipolar Disord 9:526–530, 2007

Simon MN: Generalized anxiety disorder and comorbidities such as depression, bipolar disorders and substance abuse. J Clin Psychiatry 20 (suppl 2):10–14, 2009

Spitzer RL, Endicott J, Robins E: Research Diagnostic Criteria: rationale and reliability. Arch Gen Psychiatry 35:773–782, 1978

Stordal E, Morken G, Mykletum A, et al: Monthly variations in prevalence rates of comorbid depression and anxiety in the general population at 63–65 degrees North: the Hunt study. J Affect Disord 103:273–278, 2008

Index

Page numbers printed in **boldface** type refer to tables or figures.